Self Hypnosis Loss

Heal your body and your soul. Use self-Hypnosis techniques to burn fat and lose weight. Stop the emotional eating.

Morgana Willow

Table of Contents

Introduction 4

Chapter 1 8

How to Understand Gastric Band Hypnosis

Chapter 2 16

How to lose Weight with Gastric Band Hypnosis

Chapter 3 25

Hypnosis and Meditation for Weight Loss

Chapter 4 40

Meditative Techniques

Chapter 5 49

The Concept of Overeating and Self-Hypnosis

Chapter 6 59

Burning Fat and Blasting Calories with Self-Hypnosis

Chapter 7 72

Guided Weight Loss Sessions for Hypnosis

Chapter 8..97

Tools for Reducing Body Weight

Chapter 9..115

How to use Meditation

Chapter 10 146

Dealing with Food Addiction

Introduction

If you have always struggled with your weight, or you have put on some extra pounds in the recent months or years but have not been able to get it off, you know what a difference a few extra pounds can make to how you feel, how you think, and how you interact with others. We don't want to admit that extra weight that we could be carrying is actually a problem, but the truth is, it is incredibly unhealthy.

Being overweight is not good for the body. It is also not good for the mind when you consider the implications that it can have on your self-esteem. It is important for you to consider the health effects of being overweight, and when you do, losing it is one of the only real options that you have if you want to maintain your health.

When it comes time to lose weight, you have several options. You could, for example, work out and count calories carefully. You could work toward getting liposuction or having gastric bypass surgery done. Losing weight through diet and exercise takes time and effort, and it is difficult to do well. Being able to cut out the pounds is one of the most important things that you can do when you want to make sure that your health is good. It involves a lot of effort and energy, but that is usually easier said than done.

Do you struggle with willpower? Do you struggle to stay away from the snacks and desserts no matter how hard you try to? Then you are not alone—and you can learn to overcome it. Some people might jump straight to the surgical interventions, but you can get a similar effect just by knowing how to alter your mind. When you do this enough, you can be certain that you have got that right mindset that will take you far. It all begins with knowing what you are setting out to do and how you can get past any mindset problems that you have.

One of the most important parts of getting past a problem with your relationship with food to ensure that it is healthy is being able to change your mindset, and that is what this book intends to provide for you.

Changing your mindset isn't as difficult as you might think— being able to control your mindset will help you to figure out what it is that you do need to do. When you are able to control your mindset by making sure that you take the time to influence your own actions, you should be able to also take control of your diet. The idea that you will see within this book is that through hypnosis and meditation, you can actively alter your subconscious mind so you can and will be able to take control.

Within this book, you will be provided with plenty of crucial information that you can use to ensure that your mindset is something that you can control and that through controlling your mindset, you should also be able to control everything else that goes with it. You will be able to take control of your eating patterns and your relationships with food. Now, this might sound strange or impossible, but it is true—you will be able to lose weight without having to get surgery or without having to spend hours actively counting every single calorie, and it all begins with learning to access your mindset.

After getting all of the information that you will need, from what gastric band hypnosis is and how meditation and hypnosis are actually viable options for you to lose weight, you will be guided through several guided meditations and hypnosis prompts that will help you to access your subconscious mind and help you to let go of those extra pounds without a struggle. Are you ready? Are you interested in ensuring that you get everything that you will need? Are you ready to start cutting the weight by ensuring that you have done everything possible to alter your mindset? It is all a matter of perspective—and it is time for you to get the right one.

Now, let's get started—success and a healthy relationship with food are more attainable than you think.

Chapter 1

How to Understand Gastric Band Hypnosis

If you are reading this book, you probably have some degree of an unhealthy relationship with food. Maybe you have developed a habit of emotional eating. Maybe you really enjoy eating foods that might be high in calories, and you do so without any real regard for the amount that you are eating. Perhaps you find that you have a tendency to eat more than you should be because you don't pay attention to your diet at all. No matter the reason for the imbalance of calories consumed versus burned, one thing is true: There is almost always some sort of issue with self-regulation behind obesity. Maybe you eat more but don't stay active. Maybe you eat foods that are unhealthy because they bring you joy instead of recognizing that food is fuel.

One thing is certain. However—the only tried and true method of weight loss is simple. You must eat less and exercise more. You need to burn more than you feed yourself. The body is supposed to self-regulate—you feel hungry when you need more fuel, and you are not hungry when you don't. Keep this in mind. If you look after your body the right way and make sure that you treat it well, you can ensure that the body is healthy. You can ensure that you lose weight and maintain a healthy balance.

For the most part, we are born with this innate ability to manage our weights. We are all born with the ability to ensure that we eat enough without overeating. It is instinctive to us. Have you ever seen young children overfeed themselves on their own? Most of them will naturally stop eating, even if they love the food that is in front of them when they are full. This is because they have a healthy understanding of self-regulating. It begins in infancy— breastfed babies regulate their own feeding, and we have no way to know if we are giving them enough or not enough.

Breastfeeding mothers have to trust their newborn babies to eat when they are hungry and eat enough to keep themselves filled up and with enough energy to fund their growth. At under six months of age, babies need roughly 55kcal/lb. of weight/day to grow. That means that an 8 lb. baby at birth will need 440 calories per day. How do you regulate that when you can't tell how much a baby is drinking?

They regulate themselves! They know when to stop and when to cry and look for milk. It is an instinctive reflex for them that will help them to ensure that they are getting enough to thrive. But, what happens when you are not self-regulating the right way? What if you learned early on that you have to clear your plate or you can't get up from the dinner table, even if you are already full? What if you are overeating because you have something going on?

Maybe you eat when you are bored or lonely. Maybe you eat because it is comforting for you to do so. Maybe you eat because you didn't have enough to eat as a child. Emotional eating is a huge problem that must be worked out, and that takes time. But, one thing is for sure: if you want to clean up your diet and help yourself get back to that baseline of eating to regulate yourself, you will need to start with fixing your mindset.

Gastric Band Hypnosis

When you struggle with mindset, one of the best things that you can do is ensure that you use a gastric band to manage everything.

Using a traditional gastric band is a form of weight loss that is highly invasive—you will have to cut into the upper part of the stomach, placing a band around it and physically limiting the amount of food that you can consume. This then triggers weight loss, as the stomach is restricted enough that consuming too many calories is almost impossible. But, this is also risky, invasive, and has been, as of recently, linked to several different complications after surgery, and there is always the risk of the band slipping or eroding over time.

Though the weight loss is appealing to many, the complications can make it difficult to agree to. However, in recent days, people have been becoming more interested in what is known as gastric band hypnosis—a form of hypnosis that is designed to make you believe that you have had this sort of physical procedure done and that your stomach is absolutely smaller than it was before. There is no medication or surgery used to make this work, and that allows for it to be used safely, pain-free, and effectively.

Typically, gastric band hypnosis involves two different goals. This dual-pronged approach allows you to tackle your overeating problem from two different angles to get an effective result. The first prong is taking a look at the cause of overeating in the first place. It works to figure out what kind of trauma is surrounding the act of overeating so that it can be solved. Then, after that is done, the next goal is to create that suggest that you have, in fact, had the gastric band treatment. It works to subconsciously believe that you have had your stomach size limited so that you will not eat as much. The goal is so that the body will believe that you are fuller quicker, and therefore, you will be able to cut out the calories and eat less just by virtue of the fact that you will not feel as hungry as you did before.

How Gastric Band Hypnosis Works

Gastric band hypnosis works for a simple reason: It changes your mind from the subconscious mind. Hypnosis is a method that can commonly be used to relax your mind and open yourself up to suggestions. This is important—when you are in a state of relaxation and suggestion, you can then have the hypnotist help you to guide how you feel. The state of suggestibility allows the hypnotist to start to alter what you are thinking or feeling. It will help you to figure out how everything works and to ensure that you have the confidence and behavioral changes necessary to ensure that you can commit to this lifestyle change.

Oftentimes, along with the initial hypnosis state being achieved, you will also see the teaching of self-hypnosis techniques, which will allow you to continue to enhance the work that has been done with you. Through the state of suggestibility being created, a degree of attention falling upon teaching you how to focus on yourself, and through education on nutrition and exercise, you can create that desired effect of losing weight quickly and easily.

Your mind is powerful, and the subconscious mind is responsible for most of the day-to-day habitual actions that you don't pay attention to, including what you do with your diet and exercise if you are not really paying close attention to it. Your subconscious mind will guide your decisions that you make—it influences whether you naturally reach for the ice cream or a bowl of fresh fruit and the like. When your subconscious mind struggles to make those healthier choices due to other underlying issues, such as emotional eating or having learned not to follow its own natural rhythm, you can run into some serious problems. You need to be able to take control f your subconscious to alter the habits that you have.

Taking Back Control of Your Life and Diet—One Thought at a Time

Your gastric bypass hypnosis will involve you learning to return to that state in which you do not overeat. It will help you begin to readjust your taste and your habits little by little, so you can prevent that overeating that is problematic. Through mastering these new habits, you will develop a healthier relationship with the food that you consume. Because of that, you will discover that you can make the adventure of eating that much better—you can find that you will connect better with the food that you eat and ensure that your body is healthy. Learning how to keep your body healthy is perfect, but it takes practice if you were not taught.

By starting to control yourself, you will need to access that subconscious mind. This is where your positive thinking skills will come into play. When you do this, you will be able to eliminate the problems that you run into. You will be able to work against those negative thoughts that you have and change them little by little.

However, you must be aware that this is not for everyone—the ones that have the most success in this form of hypnotherapy are those who truly want to change themselves.

The ones who are truly driven to change themselves are those who can make the most out of what they are doing at any given point in time. This isn't some magical crutch that will work like flipping a light off or on. It is a form that requires you to be well aware of what you are doing and desire to actually make that change to be successful. If you want to be able to lose weight, this can help, but only if you believe that it will. You need to align your mind with your goals to ensure that you do.

The key here is that you have to take control of your life. You will need to ensure that your life and diet are aligned well with your thoughts. To take complete control of everything, you need to have the right mindset, and you need to feel driven to make it happen for you. If you can do that, you can successfully navigate through these difficult situations. Once you have the mindset developing for yourself, you will be able to begin doing more.

You will be able to begin figuring out what it was that caused your problems with your mindset in the first place.

Chapter 2

How to lose Weight with Gastric Band Hypnosis

Now, all of this might sound incredibly compelling. But, it is only going to happen if you actually work to lose the weight and you actually want to. It seems like a fantastic option for most people, but in reality, you need to understand that it will still require work and upkeep. If you choose to utilize gastric band hypnosis, you are committing to ensuring that your mind and body are healthier just due to the fact that you will be changing your mindset and the relationship with the food that you consume. Will it work for you? The answer is a resounding maybe—but if you are committed, it will.

Within this chapter, we will look at whatever it will take for you to figure out how to lose weight with gastric band hypnosis. It is something that you will need to do carefully and deliberately, and you will need to take the time to actually try to make it work for you. But, if you know what you are doing, you can ensure that ultimately, you can and will get to that point of success. We will first go over what you can expect with your experience that you will have. This will help you know what is going to happen during the course of this book and how you can get through it all. Then, we will go over the effectiveness of gastric band hypnosis and why and how it is able to get those effects that you need. Finally, we will take a look at some of the ways that you can expect gastric band hypnosis to lead to weight loss.

What to Expect with Gastric Band Hypnosis

If you are seeing a hypnotist, you can expect your process to go pretty similarly. You will have several meetings with a hypnotherapist who will help guide you on your journey and to help you get whatever it is that you hope to achieve. You will discover that your therapist is there to help you. He or she will help by getting to know your previous attempts to lose weight. Don't feel too unnerved or uncomfortable if you are asked some questions that you would consider to be prying or nosy—your therapist wants to make sure that they are on the right page to ensure that you are actually getting the treatment that you need. They want to know about your past failures, so they can make sure that you succeed this time around.

Your therapist will help you to figure out how best to treat your weight gain so that you can start losing weight. The procedure itself is designed to make you feel like you actually got the therapy. If you go to a hypnotherapist, they may go over everything that happens in normal surgery. They may ask you to go to an actual operating room, preparing as you normally would. You will go through everything, step by step, and the therapist will slowly hypnotize you. You will be talked into that state of relaxation, and once there, the therapist will describe the process of the entire operation, step by step, from being put under to making incisions, fitting the band, and repairing the wound. You will be described to while being exposed to the normal sounds and scents of the operating room, helping to further persuade your subconscious that you are there, and it is happening.

At the same time, the therapist is likely to discuss self-confidence boosting moments as well and will work with you to get yourself into that state of relaxation. Once there, you will be able to calm down and relax. They may also teach you some self-hypnosis techniques that you can use at home as well to ensure that you are able to keep up with your weight loss.

After the therapy, you should feel calm. You should not feel any pain or discomfort—just that state of relaxation that you were in during the hypnosis. The hope is that through this process, you will start to feel fuller sooner when you are eating, allowing the therapy to work for you.

For those who overeat, it can be difficult to recognize when you are physically full, or if you are a comfort eater or a boredom eater, you may be eating regardless of physical hunger level. However, either way, learning to recognize the sensations of hunger and fullness will need to happen, and that is something that takes time.

You will be encouraged to eat mindfully and deliberately as you do— this is to hopefully create that sense of knowing how your body responds to the food that you eat and when your body is actually full.

Will it Work for Me?

Of course, this brings us to the next question—is gastric band hypnosis right for you? Many people hope that this will be their magic solution that they can use that will help them to thrive— they hope that they will be able to enjoy this therapy and magically be capable of losing their weight, but the answer is, it is up to you. While hypnotherapy can help a lot of issues, it only works if you actively want to change your habits. It is great for fixing problems related to overeating, such as feeling like it is a good emotional crutch that you can use when you are stressed, guilty, or otherwise feeling negatively. However, over time, you can work with how you take care of yourself, and you will be able to make that commitment that you needed.

Keep in mind that gastric band hypnosis is a commitment to losing weight. Just like any other commitment, it will take time and effort. It will be difficult at times, and that is okay. Ultimately, it will be your degree of commitment that will ensure that you are on the right track and ready and able to successfully make things work for you. All you will need to do is be ready to commit as much as you can. What can you tell yourself to help you to feel like you can do this? Ultimately, it will require a degree of self-confidence.

This will only work for you if you are willing and able. If you believe in the therapy process, and you trust the hypnosis that you receive, you will be more likely to successfully get through your therapy and see those results that you are looking for. You will need to approach with an open mind to get that added effect that you are looking for. When you do this, you are more likely to make those changes that you need. You will be more likely to truly absorb whatever your hypnotherapist has said to you if you believe in them and the process. This is why it is a good idea to research the therapists in your area if you go down the traditional path; you will want to make sure that you can build that rapport that you need with them, and that means being able to feel more comfortable with the people that you are around.

Ultimately, if you are someone who is dedicated and willing to keep an open mind, this form of hypnosis is incredibly powerful and can really help to make those changes that you want or need to see. If you believe in the process and you have that degree of trust with your therapist, you are much more likely to absorb the messages that you need and begin the positive changes to your lifestyle that hypnosis will encourage. It is only when you start to adopt those answers to what will be sustainable that you start to see what the right answer is. Remember, even if this is not the option for you, there is a good chance that there is an option out there for you.

How Gastric Band Hypnosis Leads to Weight Loss

Gastric band hypnosis works because it is a way that you will be able to create that weight loss that you need. As we've established, you need to have the right mindset to get the right results. Why may you ask? Simple: Our mindset is everything. Our thoughts that we have influenced our actions, and because of that, even the most unconscious thoughts become some of our worst enemies sometimes. Maybe you have a thought that you are not good enough, for example—that kind of thought would directly and actively sabotage everything that you are trying to work for.

When you think negatively, you feel bad. When you feel bad, you may fall into habits of bad eating that could be hugely problematic for you. We all have ways that we handle stress and negativity, whether it is through overeating, playing games, procrastinating, smoking, drinking, or anything else. Some people develop healthier methods of handling their stress, such as exercising.

What is your coping mechanism when things get rough? After a fight with your partner, do you run to the fridge for the carton of ice cream and a bottle of wine? If so, you might find yourself struggling with your weight before long. These are bad habits that are naturally ingrained in your mind and may have even come from how you were raised as a child. What does this mean for you? It means that you will need to find a new way to override those bad habits to fix the problem.

If you are a stress eater, very little is going to help you keep the weight off if you are constantly reaching for the ice cream and cookies after a hard day. There is a very good chance that somewhere within you, you have that habit built into your unconscious mind, meaning that the only way that you can fix the problem for yourself is to beat those bad habits

This is how hypnosis will help you to lose weight—it will work with you to ensure that as you go, you will be able to figure out what it is that you can do to fix those bad habits.

Hypnotherapy works by rewiring those habits that you have to create alternatives. Instead of reaching for the ice cream when you are stressed, for example, you could choose to go exercise instead.

Through well-crafted hypnotherapy, you could simply encourage yourself to figure out what you can do to better the situation. You could choose to intentionally choose healthier foods to eat instead of the bad ones. Or, you could choose to eat in moderation instead of anything else. There are so many ways that you can work with yourself to up your emotions and reactions.

Ultimately, as those habits are rewritten and encouraged over time, you are able to start making those lasting changes that you will need to start losing weight. When you lose weight, it becomes easier and easier for you to succeed. The good news is, as you slowly build those habits up that you want or need to have, you start seeing that you can actually reinforce them. When you realize that reaching for the bike instead of the wine is easier than you thought and you start to enjoy the processes of exercising, of eating healthily, and of how you feel as you start returning to those healthier habits that you need, you will feel better.

You will feel like you are more capable of that success that you are looking for, and you will feel more enabled than ever to get through it all. You will be more capable than ever to ensure that you would get what you were looking for: Those good habits that you will need.

The good habits that you can develop over time will help you— they will ensure that you will begin to do better. You will be more and more capable of losing the weight, little by little. You will be more and more capable of becoming the healthier individual that you want to become.

Of course, you will need to maintain the mindset as well, and that is why you will see that in the later chapters, you will discover tha

there are affirmations that can help you to stay on track. You will be given several affirmations to listen to while you drive, rest, or even sleep, which will help you to listen and absorb the messages that you are enough and that you are more than capable of losing the weight. These affirmations are meant to help you remember the habits that you want to develop and what you can do to maintain them.

So are you convinced yet? Are you interested in giving meditation and hypnosis for weight loss a try? If so, it is time to get started— the next few chapters will guide you through everything that you will need to make it work for you.

Chapter 3

Hypnosis and Meditation for Weight Loss

It all begins with an understanding of meditation and hypnosis. The truth is, the first part, getting the hypnosis that convinces you that you have had the surgery, is just the first step in this long journey.

You need to upkeep the therapy as well, and that is done primarily through the use of meditation and self-hypnosis that you can perform at home as well. These different options allow you to begin to overcome the bad habits that you have developed—they ensure that you will be able to maintain the willpower that you will need if you want to be more capable of maintaining your weight loss as well. If you know what you are doing, you should find that both meditation and hypnosis will help you immensely.

Within this chapter, you will discover several key facts that will help you to figure out how to keep your weight loss going for you. We will take a look at everything that you will need to do and why. You are looking to change your mindset, and that takes time and effort, but if you take the time, it will happen for you. We will go over just how powerful your mind is and why it has that power in the first place.

We will take a look at the routine and how it ingrains in mind. We will look at what you must do to change your mindset, and we will wrap up with an understanding of both meditation and hypnosis as influencers of the mind to create the changes that you will need.

The Power of the Mind

It all begins by looking at your mind. If you have ever attempted to lose weight before, you know that it is more than just exercising and tracking calories. While that is the simplest breakdown of what happens when you attempt to lose weight, there is more to it as well. You will need to train your mind, as well. Your mindset will change so much about how you lose weight and will help to ensure that it is a permanent loss rather than falling for that common trap of cycling between weight loss and weight gain while slowly but surely becoming heavier and heavier as you go. It is important for you to figure out how you can lose the weight little by little and stick to it— and if you want to do this, you need to make sure that your mind is in the right spot.

Excess weight is usually a sign that your mental state is not where it should be. You might be eating for stress or for comfort instead of what it is for: to sustain your body. Food is fuel, and if you fail to lose and keep off the weight, it is usually because you are failing to maintain that mindset for yourself. If you cannot convince yourself that you need to lose weight, you will never actually keep it off. If your beliefs are negative, the weight will stay on—end of the story.

Women commonly hear that they are told that they need to look a certain way—they build this expectation that they must be petite and slim in order to be attractive. But, there aren't many people that actually fit in that particular category—which means that there are a whole lot of women who think that they simply do not look very good. This is a huge problem: When you have people thinking that they are unattractive, the end result is that they do not actually feel good about themselves. Without the confidence that they would need, they cannot feel like they are beautiful. They feel bad about themselves, and what does that do?

Well, for some, they stress eat. What's it matter if they're already the wrong body type anyway? Of course, it does matter, and it is a matter of the mind. When people are confident in themselves, their appearance, and how they act, they are less likely to overeat.

Getting the right mindset for weight loss becomes the most crucial part of this journey. That's right—the mindset is more important than losing the weight itself for one very important reason: If you don't have the right mindset, you will find yourself feeling like you cannot succeed.

Changing Your Mindset

If you want to change your mindset, you might be wondering what you can possibly do. Thankfully, there are dozens of ways that you can go about fixing your mindset. There are all sorts of options that you have that will help you to craft that proper change to what your inner narrative tells you, and as you change those thoughts, you notice that your behaviors change naturally, as if directly as a result. This is perfect for you: It will ensure that you do properly get that change in mindset that you need.

How, you may be wondering? Simple: You just work on your reprogramming skills. Many of these options will exist for you through the techniques that we will discuss in the future chapters. Others are simple enough that they don't really need much of an explanation beyond what you will get here. Either way, there are changes to the mindset that can be made that will be real game-changers for you. They work to help you to love yourself, to recognize that you are in the right mindset to craft your reality the right way. It all begins with starting on the right foot.

Self-talk

The first important method that we will look at is learning to listen and change your self-talk. Your self-talk that you have within yourself matters greatly—it is with your self-talk that you can start figuring out what it is that you should be saying to yourself. It also gives you that chance to listen to how you are currently talking to yourself. What is it that you say to yourself when you think that no one else is listening? What is it that you think and feel when no one is around?

Depending upon what it is, you might find yourself thinking or feeling in very specific manners. If you speak to yourself harshly, can you really be surprised if you don't actually like the person that you are or the habits that you have?

Changing your self-talk helps to protect that inner self that you have. It helps you to ensure that the person that you are in the one that you want to be, and it honors the way that you ought to be spoken to in the first place. Stop and listen to your language.

And, when you find that you are speaking too harshly to yourself, make an active decision to change it. Only then, with that conscious effort, will you be able to change the way that you think or feel.

Rewriting your story

Another common method that people use to change their thoughts is to rewrite their own stories. When you work to be the protagonist of your story rather than the victim of life or circumstance, you have a mindset shift. The protagonist is the main character—and even when things are going rough for the main character, they normally find a way that they can change it up. They normally figure out what they can do if they want to be better for themselves, and they discover how they can possibly become that person that will be more in-tune with who they want to be.

Think about it—if you think of yourself as the main character of your story, you will realize that things work out, in the end, one way or another. You will see that the truth is that you can and will succeed if you know what you are doing. And, if you know what you are doing enough, you will realize that ultimately, you do have the ability.

Shifting to this thought will help you to stop feeling like the world is out to get you or like you are tasked with something impossible. Yes, losing weight is hard—but it is something that you can manage. Very few people out there truly cannot lose excess weight, and if you really have the weight to lose, there is probably a way that you can cut it out. All you have to do is figure out the right answer for you.

Goal-setting

Through setting goals, you can help yourself to find the direction that you need. With the right kind of attention to your own desires and actions, you can help yourself to figure out what you will need to do. When you are able to set those goals that you need, you redirect

yourself—you find a way for yourself to figure out what you are doing and how. With goals that are actually attainable, you can work with yourself. Attainable goals are those that are more nuanced than what you might initially think of. Think about it—if you have those goals that you are striving for that are larger, they are usually longer- term goals. This would be, for example, the total weight loss that you want to achieve. But, if you were to stop yourself and tell yourself that you have these shorter-term goals as well that you can follow, you can help yourself to maintain that semblance of success.

You might start by saying that you want to lose one or two pounds per week. This is a healthy to moderate amount of weight, depending on how much you have to lose and what you will do. But, having that sort of breakdown helps you to not feel so discouraged when it matters the most. Having a goal of losing a large amount of weight is fine—but it is also a long-term goal for a reason. You need to make sure that you have those shorter-term goals as well that will help you. Those shorter-term goals will give you something a bit more tangible to touch upon. They will give you that smaller thing to aim for. When you have that smaller target, you can achieve it sooner, and though it is just one small step in your journey, that still gives you the satisfaction of having succeeded in the first place, no matter how small it was.

Mindfulness

Mindfulness is a form of awareness in which you hyper-focus on what you do and how you do it. When you focus on something mindfully, you keep your focus entirely on that one thing that you are doing. It could be that you want to focus on your food and the sensation of eating. This is an important one for many undergoing this form of hypnosis—it will help you to ensure that you actually know what you are doing and help you to see the signs that you are full or done eating. When you have that understanding of when you have finished eating, you will be able to do more with yourself. You could, for example, make sure that you are done with the food that you have consumed rather than going for a clean plate if you focus on the sensation of eating itself.

Mindfulness is a wonderful way to slow yourself down as well. Some people develop a tendency to eat too quickly because they had trouble getting food when they were younger. That sort of food insecurity is difficult to get past and can lead to weight gain if you are not careful just due to eating too quickly. But, one thing is for sure: If you eat mindfully, you can find the signs that you are full and slow yourself down.

Affirmations

Affirmations are a form of kind statements that you can use to slowly and surely rewrite your mind. They are incredibly popular, and we will have an entire chapter of nothing but affirmations to help you with your weight loss journey. Nevertheless, they remain an important mention here. When it comes to making sure that you know what you need to know, you can make it happen with affirmations.

Affirmations are simple to create for yourself—they must be simple statements that assert your worth or wellbeing. When you do this the right way, you ensure that you have that common, kind expression to yourself, and that will help you to feel better. It all starts with an understanding of what it is that you want. What do you want to change how you think? Do you feel like you are worthless? Lazy?

Unimportant? Unworthy? Whatever it is that you find to be your weakness, identify it, and use that to help yourself figure out how to fix the mindset problem. When you know what it is, you create a statement that is positive about yourself. For example, imagine that you tend to overeat because you feel like food will not reject you.

This is a common form of emotional eating. If this is something that you suffer from, you might want to try statements such as "I am good enough, and I accept myself just the way that I am." Yes, you might want to lose weight, but you accept who you are. You accept that you are a person that may struggle sometimes, but you are a person nonetheless. You are good enough, and you do not need to turn to food to comfort you.

Meditation as a Mind-Changer

Meditation is a powerful tool in this all. Meditation will allow you to change your mind little by little through actually rewiring your brain. Did you know that the mindful breathing and meditations that you do can actually change the brain? Through meditation, you are able to create actual physical changes that can be noted on brain scans.

Doctors have been perplexed by this, but the truth is, when you work with your mind, you use your mind. The way that you do so also helps to reinforce positive changes that can help you to ensure that you successfully get through everything that you are doing as well.

Through knowing how to change your mind over time, you create these very real effects that help to alter the brain.

Meditation has been found to influence several key regions of the brain that are incredibly important to your general focus. It changes the left hippocampus, which is the part of your brain responsible for aiding in learning. This area of the brain helps you to remember and think and is also associated with several emotional abilities as well. In particular, it is associated with empathy, self-awareness, and emotional regulation. Through meditation, it has been found that the brain strengthens these areas, reinforcing the brain through upping the grey matter density. As you boost the grey matter in your brain, you make your brain run more effectively.

Meditation also influences the posterior cingulate. This is the part of the brain that has been connected with having a mind that is highly distractible. When your mind is distractible, you can run into all sorts of complicated issues that can make it harder for you to think or focus. However, through meditation, your area able to boost the strength of the posterior cingulate, making it strong enough to keep you on focus more. This will help you with the action of mindfulness and the ability to focus on what you do at the moment without allowing your emotions to influence your behavior.

The pons is another important part of the mind that is full of neurotransmitters that will help with the regulation of brain activity.

This is located in the center of the brain stem and helps you with sleep, physical functioning, and facial expressions.

Next, the temporoparietal junction is another crucial part of the brain that is altered through meditation. This part of the brain is responsible for the creation of empathy and compassion. In meditating, you can start to see more about the world around you.

You learn to focus on other people instead of yourself, and that can help immensely. It gives you the ability to put yourself in the shoes of someone else, which commonly reveals that things were not as bad as you may have initially thought. This is perfect for allowing you to get a good sense of perspective, which may help with emotional regulation as well.

Finally, the amygdala is influenced through meditation as well. However, unlike the other areas of the brain that we just discussed, the amygdala actually shrinks instead of grows. This is important here—the amygdala is the part of the brain that is responsible for feelings of fear and anxiety. It is the center of stress in general, and in those who meditate regularly, it tends to be smaller. In fact, even after just eight weeks of meditation practice, there is a noticeable decrease in the size of the amygdala, implying that it actually will be influenced if you know what you are doing.

Essentially, meditation is full of all sorts of good benefits that you can draw from to ensure that at the end of the day, your body and mind are working well. If you know what you are doing, you can reduce the levels of stress, have a clearer mind, and ensure that at the end of the day, you can and will provide yourself with the degree of clarity that you will need to master if you want to ensure that you are successful in your endeavors of weight loss.

This is exactly why we want to look at it as a viable option for helping you to lose weight. When you use your skills as a meditator to help yourself focus and ensure that at the end of the day, you do have the right mindset, you also naturally cause yourself to stress less as well.

You naturally influence the degree of stress that you have when you try to do something, and that matters immensely.

Hypnosis to Influence the Mind

Like meditation, hypnosis is also incredibly influential to the mind. Through mastering hypnosis, you can work with yourself to get the effect that you are looking for with weight loss. Though it can seem weird that something that you feel like you fall asleep while being hypnotized is actually changing the mind, consider this: Hypnosis is not actively turning off your brain—it is simply changing the way that your brain is functioning. You are not becoming unaware—you are becoming hyperaware. You are focusing entirely on one thing in that moment—the hypnotist, or yourself if you are performing self- hypnosis. Being able to master this allows you to become much more capable of successfully absorbing the suggestions that are made to you because your subconscious is still listening during the act of hypnosis itself.

During your trance, you shift into a different sort of brain function. During a study that looked at whether people who would be hypnotized had any sort of differences in their responses, there were several related to showing less inhibition, more engagement, and more focus on the body. Additionally, those in a hypnotic trance were also able to experience stressful thoughts without having the same sort of adverse side effects, such as higher blood pressure or sweating. It helps to allow the individual to live entirely in the moment, not unlike how it does in meditation. This makes hypnosis a similar state of mind that you would get in mindful meditation, and it follows that often, you have very similar effects of coping with.

Chapter 4

Meditative Techniques

Remember, hypnosis and meditation both require you to be relaxed so that the mind can be shifted into the right sort of mindset that you are looking for. This means that if you want to be able to follow the tactics in future chapters, you will need to look at these different hypnosis tactics that you can use.

Think of this chapter as your guide to everything that you need to know about hypnosis. If you know what you are doing, you will be able to create that added effect that you are looking for. It all begins with the induction—the ability to create the state of being entranced in the first place.

Within this chapter, you will be introduced to several different hypnotic and meditative techniques that you will be able to utilize. These will help you to ensure that at the end of the day, you can get into that trance that you will need to help you succeed. All you will need to do is ensure that you are on the right track.

Relaxation Hypnosis

When you first go to a hypnotherapist, they often tell you to relax and get comfortable—for a good reason. You need to be relaxed if you want to fall into a trance, and getting incredibly comfortable is one of the best ways that you can then use your words to suggest to someone else. Through the use of progressive relaxation, you can encourage an individual to fall into a trance, and at that point, the mind becomes open to uncomfortable. There are all sorts of suggestions that can be made to help get to that state of relaxation in the first place.

Getting comfortable is just the beginning. From there, many people will use other actions to help finish the process. You might find that you go through counting or using deep breathing to help yourself to fall into that calmer state that you will need. No matter what you need, the most important part is making sure that you are comfortable. When you can find that comfortable state, you will be able to enter the suggestibility state that will allow for the hypnotic suggestions to be made and alter your mind.

Visualization Hypnosis

Visualization hypnosis is another form of relaxation that can be used to trigger the trance while also making the suggestions that you want them to. For example, you might find yourself imagining a room that you know and are familiar with, going over every single detail in your mind. You might go over how it smells and looks. In terms of weight loss, you could go by sitting down at a table ad finding a meal that you are working through.

When you want to change the mind, you could start focusing on the positive and rewarding behaviors while also discarding the bad parts. This would be the parts such as overeating. You might imagine yourself wondering what you could do to help yourself eat less. You might feel like you are taking all of the negative energy that you have and then reject it. When you do this enough, you will begin to reject the idea of that negativity in the first place, which can help you to figure out how to keep your habits healthier as well.

You could also imagine yourself discarding those bad habits that you have or letting go of the negativity that you have allowed to rule you. No matter how you do this, you can find yourself healing yourself little by little. You can allow yourself to reject those feelings that you need to get rid of.

Breathing Hypnosis

Through breathing hypnosis methods, you can help yourself enter that state of suggestibility as well. By taking the time to go over everything yourself and controlling your breathing, you can calm yourself down just enough to enter that state of relaxation that you were aiming for.

Through controlling your breathing, you will find yourself becoming more capable of finding that success or contentment. You could find yourself calmer than ever. This makes this a wonderful method that you can use if you need to control yourself in a moment of weakness. Imagine that you are really stressed out, and you're someone that will tend to stress eat. If you stop and use a breathing exercise, you can bring yourself back down to that state of calmness that you need.

Hypnotic Logic

When you are in a state in which you are suggestible, you can start to implement hypnotic logic. This works because, during the trance state, you are going to be susceptible to suggestion. You will also take statements literally when you hear them. If you ask someone if they can stand up, they will respond by answering yes instead of actually getting up. If you know what you are doing, you can begin to implement this sort of logic with yourself as well.

You can tell yourself that you can lose weight because you know that you are successful or because you know that you are determined. By shifting away from saying that you want to lose weight to saying in that state that you can lose the weight, you will naturally absorb that statement to mean what you want it to. You will then begin to recognize that you can and will be able to lose the weight—you just have to work through it.

Body Scan Meditation

When it comes to meditative techniques, one of the best things that you can do is work through body scans. This is perfect if you are trying to practice self-hypnosis. It allows you to focus on the sensations within your body, little by little so that you can be certain that you are calm. If you need to keep yourself from overeating, this can be a fantastic option—scanning your body can help you to figure out how you feel at the moment. Are you eating? A quick body scan can help you to figure out how much to continue eating, as well as help you to identify when you are all full. It can also help you to become more in touch with how you feel as you get through it all.

You can also use body scanning to help yourself get into a hypnotic trance as well. Through carefully paying attention to each and every sensation within your body, you will eventually work yourself into that trance sensation that you were looking to get into in the first place.

This is a technique that you can also use with other meditative and hypnotic techniques as well.

Reframing Meditation

Reframing meditations allow you to change the perspective that you took on a certain experience, and they can be especially useful if you are tarrying to get yourself to change a habit. They are usually done as a sort of metaphor to help create a connection between two things that ought to be done. For example, if you love to quilt, but you need to get yourself up and active, you can start to imagine your body as a quilt that needs to be created. You compare the act of quilting to the act of creating the weight loss that you need. This helps to create that expectation and understanding that this is a

slow-going process, and it will take time. For example, you could say, "Losing the weight is like creating a quilt. Every day, you work on one patch at a time, until eventually, you can put them all together. At first, you don't have a quilt that you can use, but little by little, your quilt becomes closer and closer to being completed, and eventually, it is done. After all of your effort and energy, you see the whole picture for yourself, and you can use it once and for all."

This sort of reframing allows you to take something that might be difficult to cope with, such as losing weight and make it seem like something that is desirable. Let's face it—if you are here reading this book, you've probably struggled with weight loss in the past. You might have certain hang-ups about trying to lose weight now. But, if you compare the weight loss process to something that is actually tolerable, you will find that it is not nearly as bad as you might have initially thought.

Affirmation Meditation

Affirmation meditations are all about shifting your mindset from something negative to something positive. Imagine that you are currently suffering from body dysmorphia—you think that you are bigger than you actually are. If you have this sort of negativity about yourself and hate how you look, and that is actively becoming a detriment to your weight loss process, then you can work against it by figuring out how to correct those negative thoughts. By shifting to a mindset of positivity, telling yourself what you should be thinking, you should be able to change up how you engage. Think about it— you could tell yourself that you are beautiful in several different ways. You can tell yourself that you are worthy of love, that you do not need to consume food to feel good, and other statements that will help you to shift to that positive mindset that you need.

Through creating the affirmations and repeating them as your own meditation, your mind starts to accept them, and little by little, you realize that you are more than capable of successfully navigating through these situations. You will be able to change those negative thoughts to positive ones, so they stop dragging you down and making it impossible for you to succeed.

Meditation Mantras

Meditation mantras are similar to affirmations, but instead of a series of statements, you focus on one word or concept. Your mantra is a single word that you repeat to yourself instead of a whole phrase.

While affirmations are meant to change your mindset, a mantra is meant to bring you that degree of focus that you need. It is meant to help you to ensure that you bring yourself back to your center.

Imagine that you are getting close to breaking one of the new habits that you set up for yourself—with a mantra, you could remind yourself to re-center yourself and keep yourself on track. This is perfect for those moments of weakness, and we all have them at one point or another. Your mantra becomes that central point that you can turn to when you feel overwhelmed or like those negative thoughts are going to take everything over.

Guided Meditation

Finally, guided meditations are those in which you follow along with a meditation that is narrated by someone else. As you get to the future chapters, you are looking at a series of guided meditations that are meant to help you conquer that negativity that you might have deeply ingrained in yourself. These meditations are meant to exist with a narrator or hypnotist carefully and gently guiding you into a state of relaxation and guiding you on the entire meditation to get to the end result that you wanted.

The meditation itself is what you will focus on as you go through the chapters. It is the part that you will be entranced by, and it will help you to create or evoke certain images that you can use to ensure that you are successful in getting to your end result.

Chapter 5

The Concept of Overeating and Self-Hypnosis

Are you ready to start preventing yourself from overeating? This hypnosis prompt is meant to relax you into convincing your subconscious mind that your stomach has been surgically shrunk so that you cannot eat as much food to prevent yourself from overeating the foods around you. If you want to lose weight but do not want invasive surgery, this is one of the best ways that you can make it happen. This may be something that is a bit gorier than you want to hear, as it is effectively a visualization meditation that is meant to walk you through the surgery, but it is meant to be effective.

Are you ready? If so, make sure that you are settled down somewhere that is quiet and relaxing. Traditionally, it would be done in a staged operating room, but lying on your bed can work as well.

Gastric Band Hypnosis Script

You breathe in... And out... And in... And out... As you do, you find yourself relaxing more and more. Close your eyes and take a deep breath. As you take a deep breath through your nose, you realize that you can smell the scent of sterile alcohol all around you. It smells like someone has doused the whole room in rubbing alcohol to clean it, and you can smell the sharp scent of stainless steel all around you. You breathe in... and you smell gloves on someone's hand.

You can see a very bright light right above you. It is almost impossible for you to see past the brightness above you, even if you want to. The rest of the room beyond the light is dark. You can hear voices talking about preparation for surgery. You feel a hand touch yours, and when you turn, you see a person in teal scrubs, with a face mask and a bandana over their hair to keep it in place.

"We are going to begin the procedure. Are you ready?" You nod your head to the person.

"You are going to feel a small pinch as we insert the IV, okay?" The person next to you says. "And then, you will count to ten and fall asleep."

You nod your head again. You feel perfectly at ease where you are. You are not worried at all as you are there. You know that you are in great hands and that they will take care of you just how you need to. You know that they are going to help you to be put on a path toward a healthier life, and you are ready to embrace it.

You feel the pinch in your arm, followed by cool liquid flowing through your vein right in the area that it was placed. You feel pressure on your arm where they tape the IV into place so you cannot knock it off. You start to feel a bit heavy and floaty as whatever is in the IV flows into your body.

Then, they put a mask over your mouth and nose. It is big and cool, and it presses into your skin around your face. It is pushed a bit harder than you expected to create a tight seal, and then you hear them instruct you to count backward from ten to calm yourself down.

"Ten..." you begin, feeling a bit dizzy. You are relaxed.

"Nine..." You are feeling heavier now than you did before like you are sinking onto the operating table.

"Eight..." You are getting even more tired than you were before, and your eyelids are getting heavy. You can't keep them open any longer.

"Seven..." The whole body feels heavy and like it can't move. "Six..." You can barely say a word at that point.

"Five..." And the whole world fades away. You can't move anymore. You are stuck where you are, and you feel at ease.

You are in complete and utter relaxation at the moment. You are not afraid or worried. You are not in pain or uncomfortable. Your eyes are closed, but you are aware that the people around you are talking.

"We must make the incision," you hear one of them say, and suddenly, you feel pressure on your stomach. You feel just pressure

—no pain. You can feel it in several different places on your body. You feel it up near your stomach, then a few more places as well. "We are putting in four incisions so we can get the band in," the surgeon states. "We will be able to do so with this laparoscopic camera."

You feel tugging and pressure again as they situation their camera where it needs to be. "Now that it is there, we can see what we are doing. Do you see the stomach there?"

You can hear some people state their agreement and acknowledgment.

"Good. We will be putting a band around this part right here," he stated. "We will be separating that upper part of the stomach from the lower part so the patient cannot eat as much food at any point in time. We are making the stomach's volume smaller so the patient must eat less and, therefore, will lose weight. Any questions?"

Someone else starts to speak. "Will it hurt?"

"It might be uncomfortable for a few days after the procedure, but they should be perfectly comfortable. We do this laparoscopically, so there is less pain during recovery. It should be a simple procedure.

Any more questions?"

There is silence, so the surgeon goes back to work. You can feel pressure in your torso. It is not uncomfortable—just foreign. The surgeon works with small tools that allow them to access your stomach without opening you up as much, and that allows them to treat you easier.

"We have the band situated now," the surgeon says after a few minutes. They didn't take long to find the right spot at all. And, as they do so, they secure the band around your stomach. You feel pressure around your stomach as its capacity for food has been dramatically reduced.

"And it's done." The surgeon pulls back, and you feel a strange tugging in your stomach in four places, and then settling. The little tools have been removed from within you. You can vaguely smell the scent of blood among the stainless steel and sterile alcohol, and you feel pressure on top of all four incision sites. You can feel that they are doing this to get the bleeding taken care of.

You are perfectly relaxed, and though you can feel pressure, you are not in pain. You are aware of the fact that you can feel the strange

pressure on your stomach that has cut the amount of space that you can fill in half. You can feel that you can no longer eat as much, and you recognize that this is a direct result of the band being placed there for you. You are directly aware of the fact that you have gotten that band situated and that your stomach's volume is now dramatically reduced, and that you will not be able to eat as much.

"The patient will only be able to consume roughly 1 cup of food now. A normal stomach holds up to 4. But it looks like we are done. It is time to take the patient to recovery."

And then, you are unaware of anything else.

You wake up slowly, feeling groggy and slow. You feel heavy, but you are still not in any pain. You are comfortable and ready to go forward. You are ready to go.

"Don't move so much," someone says next to you, and you see a nurse there, taking care of you and trying to get you comfortable. "Are you in pain?"

You shake your head no. You are quite comfortable, though your stomach feels much smaller.

"Good. We need to get you to eat to ensure that the surgery has worked. Are you ready?"

You nod your head, and they hand you a small cup. "It's full of broth," they tell you, and you nod again. You take a sip. Your stomach feels uncomfortably full already. You realize that you cannot consume nearly as much as you could before. It is strange, but you see that ultimately, you have no choice. You need to eat less so you can lose weight.

Over the next few weeks, you can only consume a very small amount of food at any point in time. You should be very careful with how much you eat, and if you overeat, you will find yourself vomiting.

You will find yourself struggling to get through the food. You will find yourself being unable to keep as much in your stomach.

At first, it is recommended that you only eat liquid foods so that you can adjust to your stomach being this new size. It is not painful—just different. You will not feel pain—just different. You will feel pressure, and you will feel that your stomach is no longer the size that it used to be. You will feel that you are no longer going to be as hungry. You can't be hungry when there isn't as much room in your stomach anymore. From here on out, portion control is everything. Portion control will keep you healthy, and it will keep you able to eat as much as you should be. It will regulate out your diet and make sure that you will only consume just as much as you needed.

You breathe in... And out... Your stomach feels tighter. It feels smaller.

You breathe in... And out... You realize that you only drank half of your broth before you were full and no longer able to have anymore.

You breathe in... And out... And you realize that you are on your way to taking back control of your own weight and life once and for all.

You breathe in... And out... And you are feeling more relaxed.

You are told that you are allowed to go home but to take it easy on the food for the next few days. You are discharged quickly with no complications, and you are free to go home.

When you get home, you are not in any pain. You never feel any pain. Just pressure. You never feel yourself getting hurt. You just feel that you are fuller much quicker. Every time, after just a few bites, you will start to get full. Every time you drink, you only drink a few drinks as well.

You feel great. You feel at ease. You feel more comfortable in your own body as you realize that you are on track to being healthy.

You breathe in. You breathe out. And you feel comfortable.

It is time to start waking up now. You breathe in... And out... And in... And out... And you realize that you are on track to the life that you want.

Breathe in... And out... And in...

And out...

Repeat to yourself:

I am capable of eating less. I will eat less.

I will not be able to eat nearly as much as I did before. I am going to lose weight.

I have a gastric band on my stomach.

I will only be able to eat a small amount of food at any given time, and I will eat it slowly and carefully.

I have a gastric band on my stomach.

I will only be able to eat a little bit at a time, and that's okay. I have a gastric band on my stomach.

I am going to be the person that I want to be.

Chapter 6

Burning Fat and Blasting Calories with Self-Hypnosis

Self-hypnosis is a powerful tool that you can use in moments of weakness. When you can remind yourself of just how powerful it is to burn your fat, working out, and reminding yourself to exercise more often, you will realize that you are capable of succeeding. You can burn that fat by remembering that you need to move. But, if you aren't motivated to get exercising, how are you supposed to keep yourself on track? What are you going to do if you are always making excuses for yourself?

When you do this the right way, you will be able to keep yourself motivated and push yourself forward. By self-hypnotizing, you can motivate yourself to keep moving forward. You will be able to remind yourself of all of the reasons that you will need to get through everything. You will help yourself figure out how you can stay on track with what you are doing and how you can continue to burn the fat to get the weight off.

Ultimately, losing weight is all about figuring out how to balance out burning calories with how many you consume. Losing weight is all about making sure that you have less in your diet than you need so that you are burning fat in your body to help continue to run your body. Maintaining weight is when you want to eat only the foods that you will need. However, if you are not exercising, you will not be getting a fully healthy body that you will need. You have to make sure that you are burning calories one way or another, and you also have to make sure that you are providing yourself with time and energy for your body to move and be active as well. When you do this the right way, you should be able to figure out what you are doing, and you should be able to get those results you are looking for.

To use self-hypnosis, all you have to do is walk yourself through relaxing to the point that you will be able to get those results that you are looking for. You want to make sure that you are walking yourself through how you can get to that same state of relaxation that a hypnotist would normally do for you.

When it comes to trying to self-hypnotizing, you have a few options. Some people choose to read their own scripts, but they are typically more effective and passive when you are listening rather than reading. For this reason, you want to try to locate some prompts that will help you.

Within this script that you will be provided, you will find yourself becoming motivated to work out more. You will be finding yourself passively taught that what you need to do above all else is to figure out how you can better yourself. You will find that you are capable of achieving that weight loss, even if you think that you are not.

This prompt is all about maintaining your willpower and helping to keep you on track. If you want to lose weight, you need to have the drive to do so, and that requires you to work through these processes. Are you ready? As with the other meditation prompts, they should not be utilized during driving or other activities for maximum effect. Listening to them as you settle down is one of the best options for you. You want to ensure that you are somewhere that you can completely relax and allow the script to kick in and create the desired intended effect, and when you figure out how to do that, you will find yourself succeeding.

Self-Hypnosis Prompt

Settle down on your bed or chair and get comfortable. You should be somewhere that is perfectly relaxing for you. You shouldn't have any distractions present, and you should feel at peace where you are. As you relax, allow your eyes to begin to close. You can be as comfortable as possible. Don't worry about relaxation and it will come. Allow yourself to sit, completely passively. Don't try to force it or try to focus too hard. Simply sit and be comfortable.

Take in a deep breath, and then breathe it out. Breathe in through your nose, feeling the air chilling your nostrils as you pull it in, and then exhale it when you try to release it all. Breathe in and breathe out. In and out. In and out. As you breathe out, you should feel the air escaping your lips in an O shape, and as you do, you should feel yourself relaxing further.

With every breath in, you feel your body nourishing itself with oxygen, and with every breath out, you feel your body purifying itself, releasing the waste that it no longer needs. Sit there and enjoy the breathing process and watch as soon it feels that your chest rises on its own and then exhales on its own. Your body is capable of giving you what you need. Your body will breathe on its own.

You trust your body to give you the air that you will need to live, and you trust it to breathe out the toxins that you need to remove. You allow your body to regulate itself, and you allow your breathing to run itself.

As you breathe, you imagine the stress and tension within yourself, gathering in your lungs. It is carried through your blood and released into the lungs, just like the air that you breathe.

The stress and tension arrive in your lungs, and you exhale it out, just like the carbon dioxide that your body tries to rid itself of.

You breathe in and out again. You feel stronger. You feel better. You feel more capable of success. You feel relaxed. You feel like

62

you are at ease where you are. As you do this, breathing in and out, you realize that you are in complete control of your body. You can change your breathing if you want to, but your body will naturally gravitate toward what it knows that you need. You know that if you

breathe faster, you can—but you might start to feel lightheaded. If you breathe slower than you need, you might start to feel like you don't have enough oxygen. You know that you are in control of your breathing, but usually, you know that it is best to let your body control your breathing itself.

Your body controls a lot of needs by itself, working on its own to change how you think, feel, and breathe. It controls how it regulates itself. Your body is very aware of everything that you are going to need to do. It is capable of controlling itself in many different ways. It is capable of making sure that you eat just enough and just the right foods if you listen to it. It is capable of ensuring that you are perfectly healthy. It is capable of ensuring that you are eating enough food and making sure that you get the right ones. It will drive you to get moving if you need to—it will make you want to get exercise if you know how to listen to it.

Your body naturally will tell you what you need, how you need it, and how to get it if you listen to it—but you have to listen. Just like with breathing, you can take control of your body's actions as well. You can choose to eat things that your body wasn't initially looking for.

You can choose to drink things that may not be very healthy for you because you like them. You can choose to sit down instead of going out to enjoy nature and explore the outdoors. You can choose to override those basic needs that you have so that you can be the healthiest that you can be.

When you do this the right way, you should be capable of getting to that point of success. This means that you need to listen to your body.

You breathe in and out... And in... And out... And you can feel your body relaxing. You can feel your body wanting to naturally do what you will need to make sure that you are healthy. You will be able to figure out how best to listen to yourself.

You feel more relaxed than ever right now. You feel like you are entirely capable of getting through the processes that you need. You

feel like you are able to drift more and more. You feel like you are sinking into your bed where you sit, and you feel ready to stay there.

You imagine yourself looking in a mirror. As you are there, you can see yourself. That part of you is yourself. That person that you see right there is the part of you that wants you to listen. You see yourself there, and you can see the look of defeat on your face. You can see the look of depression. You can see the look of being stuck right there. You do this and see that you have been silencing this part of your body. You do this and see that you have been telling yourself not to listen to the part of you that knows best. You do this and see that you are in a position to not be able to get what you need. You are actively hurting yourself by not listening to what your body is trying to tell yourself.

You can see that reflection of you, and you realize that it is the part of you that you needed to listen to more than ever. That is the part of you that wanted to be healthy—the part of you that wanted to ensure that you would be comfortable in your body. You find yourself gazing into your sad eyes, wondering what happened. What caused you to bury this part of you behind so much? What made you step away from the person that you were before, and what made you decide to suppress this person? The answer is there if you know what to listen for. You were indulgent.

Your indulgence was harmful. Your indulgence buried a part of you away so far that you felt like you would never be able to get it back. Your indulgence buried yourself behind the person that you became: Unhealthy and unable to get through everything.

That's right... there is a part of you that was actively sabotaging yourself. That part of you wanted to indulge in whatever made you happy—it wanted you to be the person that it wanted you to be without looking at what you would need.

And now, you have the opportunity to confront that part of yourself. You look down at yourself, and you realize that you are the part that has pushed that healthy part away. You are the part of yourself that caused your problems, and that means that you are the part of yourself that caused your problems, and that means that you are the only one that can fix the problem.

You must make sure that you are taking the time to better yourself. You must be willing to let go of those long-lost desires. You must be willing to get past that person that you were so that you can still lose the weight.

It is now that you will need to start making choices. You look at that part of yourself that was pushed away and silenced for so long. That is the part of yourself that was unable to be the person that you wanted to be. That is the part of yourself that knew what you needed all along. You know that you have to do something to fix the problem

—but you are unsure of what you need to do in the first place.

You must choose to make a decision now. Do you choose to listen to that part of you that knows how to lead you and how to ensure that you are the person that you want to be? Do you choose to listen to the person who can guide you to where you need to be? Do you choose to reach out and embrace that person in front of you? Or do you choose to stay where you are without making any changes?

The person in front of you, that part of yourself reaches out a hand for help. That person reaches out to ask you to listen. You beg yourself to listen. That part of you is pleading with you. "Please let me guide our body," you tell yourself. "Please let me get us outside. Please let me get us moving and active. Please let me get us healthy. We can't live like this forever. I will help, I promise, just believe me…"

You have to actively make a decision. You have to look at that person as a part of you that is a not threat; that part of you is not your enemy. That part of you is not trying to hurt you. That part is actively begging for you to embrace it. That part of you has been rejected for far too long, and your healing and your journey toward weight loss cannot begin until you take that part of you back.

You look at yourself, and you realize that you have been making a huge mistake. You realize that you've been actively causing yourself problems that must be fixed at some point. You realize that you've been making it impossible for you to do anything at all and that you will need to figure out how you can better your situation. You will need to do whatever it will take for you to lose weight and feel more confident in yourself, and that requires you to acknowledge something.

You must acknowledge that you were wrong. You must acknowledge that so far, you have been trying to tell yourself to do things that are not going to help you. You must see that ultimately, the harm that you have and are experiencing is because you have chosen not to be the person that you should be.

Every unhealthy habit that you have is not because of this person that you have suppressed—it is because you chose to ignore that person. You chose this, and now you must make it happen. You must fix the problem once and for all.

You look at yourself and take your hand. You reach out to that part of yourself that is so defeated and embrace your hand. You pull yourself closer until you are hugging yourself tightly.

You must be willing and able to apologize to yourself—you must be willing and able to remind yourself that you were the problem. You must be willing to see that your own choices were what caused all of these issues in the first place and that you will need to acknowledge that the only person that can fix the problems at this point is yourself. You can choose to make active choices to change your habits.

You apologize to yourself. You tell yourself that you cannot keep fighting so much. "I'm sorry," you tell yourself. "I'm sorry that I've left you to get hurt. I'm sorry that you've been rejected for so long.

I'm sorry that I've tried to do everything in my power to ignore and forget about you. It's not fair that I pushed you away. It's not fair that I made those unhealthy choices and that I tried to bury you deep within myself. I hurt you, and that's not fair. I'd love to include you in my life. I'd love to give you that control again. Please take back your role.

Please regulate what we need so that we can heal. It's time for me to love myself the way that I deserve to be loved—and that means loving my whole self, not just the parts that are easy. It's not easy to be healthy... It's not always easy to meet all of my needs, but I know that you are there to help me.

The only way that we can do this is if we work together, and we become one person, interested in healing and interested in being the whole person that I know we can be." You apologize to yourself. You must imagine yourself becoming at peace with yourself. You must find yourself feeling like you are healing. You must embrace that to be healthy, you must listen to your body. Your body will tell you exactly what it is that you need. Your body will tell you how you can ensure that you are healthy. It will guide you. It will make sure that you have exactly what you need and all you have to do is listen. Embrace yourself. Embrace your whole self. Don't let yourself feel hated any longer. Don't let yourself suppress who you are anymore. Embrace who you are and acknowledge that you have that control. Acknowledge that you can be healthier.

And, feel proud that you made the mature decision. Remind yourself that you have made a choice that is not easy, but it is the right one.

You breathe in, and you breathe out. You breathe in... And out...

And you feel a newfound sense of peace. You feel at ease. You know that you have to listen to your body, and if you do, your body will guide you. You know that your body will try to get you up and moving, and you know that you must follow it. You can begin healing as you listen to yourself. You can see that you are the person that you want to become. You can let go of those foods that are unhealthy and choose flavorful, enjoyable, healthier options.

Unhealthy food will no longer taste as good. In fact, it will be rejected by you more often than not.

You will realize that you get true joy following along with what you need. You will find exercise enjoyable. You will find more joy in being able to consume healthier foods. You will find yourself working better than ever, and all you have to do is make sure that you stick to what you need. All you have to do is continue to follow yourself with what you will need, and everything else will come easily.

Now... Take another deep breath in... And out... And feel the joy that you are more connected to yourself than you have ever been. And, as you awaken, allow yourself to continue to follow yourself and follow your own body's cues so you can be the healthiest person that you can be.

Chapter 7

Guided Weight Loss Sessions for

Hypnosis

Losing weight with hypnosis works a bit like the other change with hypnosis will. However, it's essential to know the step by step process so that you accurately recognize what to expect during your weight loss journey with the support of hypnosis. Generally, there are about seven steps that are involved in weight loss using hypnosis.

- The initiative is once you plan to change

- The second step involves your sessions

- The third and fourth are your changed mindset and behaviors

- The fifth step involves your regressions

- The sixth is your management routines

- The seventh is your lasting change.

To give you a far better idea of what each of those parts of your journey seems like, allow us to explore them in greater detail below.

In your initiative toward achieving weight loss with hypnosis, you've got to make a decision that you desire change, which you're willing to undertake hypnosis to vary your approach to weight loss. At now, you recognize you would like to reduce, and you've got been shown the likelihood of losing weight through hypnosis. You'll end up feeling curious, hospitable, trying something new, and a touch bit skeptical about whether this is often actually getting to work for you. You'll even be feeling frustrated, overwhelmed, or maybe defeated by the shortage of success you've got seen using other weight loss methods, which can be what leads you to hunt out hypnosis within the first place.

At this stage, the simplest thing you'll do is practice keeping an open and curious mind, as often this is how you'll set yourself up for fulfillment when it involves your actual hypnosis sessions.

Your sessions account for stage two of the method. Technically, you're getting to move from stage two through to step five several times over before you officially enter stage six. Your sessions are the stage where you engage in hypnosis, nothing more, and zip less. During your sessions, you would like to take care of your open mind and stay focused on how hypnosis can assist you. If you're struggling to remain open-minded or are still skeptical about how this might work, you'll consider switching from absolute confidence that it'll help to possess a curiosity about how it'd help instead.

Following your sessions, you're first getting to experience a changed mindset. Often this is where you begin to feel much more confident in your ability to reduce and in your ability to stay the load off. At first, your mindset should be shadowed by doubt, but as you still use hypnosis and see your results, you'll realize that you simply can create success with hypnosis. As these pieces of evidence started to point out up in your own life, you'll find your hypnosis sessions becoming even more powerful and even more successful.

In addition to a changed mindset, you're getting to start to ascertain modified behaviors. They'll be smaller initially, but you'll find that they increase over time until they reach the purpose where your expressions reflect precisely the lifestyle you've got been getting to have. The simplest part about these changed behaviors is that they're going not to feel forced, nor will they desire you've got had to encourage yourself to urge here: your changed mindset will make these changed behaviors incredibly easy for you to settle on.

As you continue performing on your hypnosis and experiencing your changed mind, you'll find that your behavioral changes grow more significant and more effortless every single time.

Following your hypnosis and your experiences with changed mindset and behaviors, you're likely getting to experience regression periods.

Regression periods are characterized by periods where you start to interact in your old mindset and behavior once more. This fact happens because you've got experienced this old mindset and behavioral patterns numerous times over that they still have deep roots in your subconscious. The more you uproot them and reinforce your new behaviors with consistent hypnosis sessions, the more success you'll have in eliminating these old behaviors and replacing them entirely with new ones.

Anytime you experience the start of a regression period, you ought to put aside a while to interact during a hypnosis session to assist you in shifting your mindset back to the state that you want and wish it to be in.

Your management routines account for the sixth step, and that they inherit place after you've got adequately experienced a big and lasting change from your hypnosis practices. At now, you're not getting to got to schedule as frequent hypnosis sessions because you're experiencing such significant changes in your mindset.

However, you'll still want to try to hypnosis sessions regularly to make sure that your mindset remains changed, which you are doing not revert into old patterns. Sometimes, it can take up to 3-6 months or longer with these consistent management routine hypnosis sessions to take care of your changes and stop you from experiencing a big regression in your mindset and behavior.

The final step in your hypnosis journey goes to be the step where you encounter lasting changes. At now , you're unlikely to wish to schedule hypnosis sessions any more.

You ought to not got to believe hypnosis in the least to vary your mindset because you've got experienced such significant changes already, and you do not end up regressing into old behaviors. Thereupon being said, you'll find that from time to time, you would like to possess a hypnosis session to take care of your changes, particularly when an unexpected trigger may arise, which will cause you to require to regress your behaviors. These sudden changes can happen for years following your successful changes, so staying on top of them and counting on your excellent coping method of hypnosis is vital because it will prevent you from experiencing a significant regression in life.

Encourage Healthy Eating Using Hypnosis

As you undergo using hypnosis to support you with weight loss, there are a couple of ways in which you're getting to do so. One of the methods is to specialize in weight loss itself. Differently, however, is to specialize in topics surrounding weight loss. For instance, you'll use hypnosis to assist you to encourage yourself to eat healthy while also helping discourage yourself from unhealthy eating.

Practical hypnosis sessions can assist you in bust cravings for foods that are getting to sabotage your success while also helping you are feeling more drawn to creating choices that are getting to assist you effectively reduce.

Many people will use hypnosis to vary their cravings, improve their metabolism, and even help themselves acquire a taste for eating healthier foods. You'll also use this to assist and encourage you to develop the motivation and energy to truly prepare healthier meals and eat them so that you're more likely to possess these healthier options available for you. If cultivating the motivation for cooking and eating healthy eating has been problematic for you, this sort of hypnosis focus is often incredibly helpful.

Using Hypnosis to Encourage Healthy Lifestyle

In addition to helping you encourage yourself to eat healthier while discouraging yourself from eating unhealthy foods, you'll also use hypnosis to assist and encourage you to form healthy lifestyle changes. This way will support you with everything from exercising more frequently to learning more active hobbies that support your wellbeing generally.

You may also use this to assist you in eliminating hobbies or experiences from your life, which will encourage unhealthy dietary habits in the first place.

For instance, if you tend to scoff once you are stressed, you would possibly use hypnosis to assist you in navigating stress more effectively so that you're less likely to scoff once you are feeling stressed. If you tend to eat once you are feeling emotional or bored, you'll use hypnosis to assist you in modifying those behaviors, too.

Hypnosis is often wont to change virtually any area of your life that motivates you to eat unhealthily or otherwise neglect self-care to the purpose where you're sabotaging yourself from healthy weight loss. It truly is an incredibly versatile practice that you simply can believe, which will assist you with weight loss, also as assist you with creating a healthier lifestyle generally. With hypnosis, there are countless ways in which you'll improve the standard of your life, making it an incredibly useful practice for you to believe. You'll use hypnosis to support yourself with weight loss, also as improving your wellbeing overall.

The Right State of Mind

Find a quiet place to take a seat or lie for complete relaxation, then breathe and concentrate. Notice that the air tides in through your nostrils and the way your belly buzzes to the utmost and gently falls back to your spine as you exhale. Allow gravity to carry you securely in situ. Breathe as naturally as you'll. Don't force your breathing and notice if your breath is quick or slow and steady.

As you inhale, accept gratitude and let warmth fill your lungs. Consider the items you're grateful for. Consider something that creates you are feeling happy and peaceful. Tell yourself, "I am thankful to be alive. I'm secure and safe. I'm confident and pure." concentrate on your heart now. As you say these words to yourself, feel them deep within you.

Give these statements positive energy and feed them amorously. "I love myself; I can do anything I put my mind to. I trust that my brain, body, and soul are capable of providing me with what I desire most in life."

Breathe in now and fill your mind and soul amorously and heat. Imagine as you inhale that there's a radiant light that fills your lungs before rapidly escaping your body. This light gives your patience, it gives you strength, and it provides you with the ambition and motivation to tackle the barriers that substitute your way. Exhale naturally and see as your body becomes heavier. With every breath that flows out, abandoning of negative thoughts; push those thoughts aside. You're ok, and you'll do that. You're loved. You're special. Exhale and release all of the strain that holds you back now.

What people believe and what you think are two various things. Say this far, "I believe myself."

Count your breaths now. As you inhale, breathe together with your belly and count. One, two, three, four, and five. Once you are abandoning this breath, confirm it's steady and slow. Exhale, two, three, four, five. You're accepting this positive light to vibrate through your entire being. You're letting go of all the negativity that holds you back. Inhale one, two, three, four.

Exhale one, two, three, four. And inhale for one, "I am happy," two, "I am strong," three, "I am kind," four, "I am brave," five, "I am driven to succeed." exhale now. You're counting your breath from one to 5 slow and steady.

Positivity embraces you now; you are feeling light and in complete control. Nothing can disturb you; nothing can bring you down; you're perfect the way you're. Repeat this step until you're able to watch your thoughts flow in and out.

Bring focus to your inner thoughts now. What pops into your mind? If you've got any negative thoughts, allow them to be there as long as they need to be without judging them. Watch them, then let them go. With every in-breath, notice your thoughts enter without judgment. These thoughts are neither positive nor negative. Once you exhale, just abandoning all hostility and anger you would possibly be holding. Let it escape into the universe and inhale, one, two, three, four, five; you're accepting all honesty and trust within yourself that you simply can make it through anything.

"I am resilient. I'm beautiful. I'm a pacesetter ."

If you notice any negative thoughts, just see them and replace them with positive, self-loving thoughts.

Breaking Barriers

Make sure that you simply are during a place where you're completely comfortable and cannot be disturbed for a minimum of thirty minutes. Have the space you're inset to a comforting temperature and confirm that the lights are low. Adjust your body so that your shoulders are relaxed, your arms are lying on either side of you, and your palms face the ceiling. You would like to become as comfortable and relaxed as you'll so that your focus isn't on your body but the meditation. Gently close your eyes and take a deep breath inward until you do not inhale. Exhale slowly and steadily so that all of the air escapes your lungs. Repeat these two more times.

Notice how your mind and body are relaxing into this guided exercise now. Breathe naturally now and convey your attention to your breath. Notice because the air fills your lungs and escapes as quickly because it entered. Breathing are some things we do a day that we frequently deem granted. It's one of the various gifts that life gives us. Just be mindful of this moment you're in immediately. Don't be concerned if your mind wanders; that's natural. There are no wrong thanks to doing that. Put trust in yourself that directly, you're not performing; you do not need to be perfect.

Bring your attention to your body and your weight now. Visualize in your mind what you appear as if and check out not to judge yourself too harshly. You're who you're, regardless of what you look as if or how you are feeling that. Erase the strain and negativity from your mind; just be present with yourself immediately.

Say to yourself

"I am beautiful. I'm strong. I can do that. I will be able to reduce, and that I won't let anyone or anything substitute my way. The sole opinion I will be able to accept is what I feel and feel about myself. At this moment and in my future moments, I think that I'm beautiful just the way that I'm ."

Let your breath suck these thoughts altogether and have your mind believe everything you tell yourself as if it had been your last wish on Earth.

As you visualize your weight immediately, I might, such as you to imagine that you are at the start of a race. There are people a bit like you're competing for fulfillment.

Say to yourself

"I got this. I will be able not to hand over. I will be able to succeed, and that I will make it to the finishing line. I will be able to conquer my fears and overcome every obstacle that stands in my way."

In the background, you hear a teacher shout, "Ready, get set..." Bring your awareness to your breath again. Inhale deeply, and as you inhale, get yourself fully committed and prepared to require your initiative toward losing weight. "Go!" exhale and visualize your feet, taking that first, second, and third breakthrough. Feel the pressure of your body depress on your legs and carry you forward. You realize this is often hard, but you do not hand over. You still jog ahead. Repeat this – "I know I can, I do know I can, I do know I can. I won't hand over; I can do that ."

You are now arising to a bicycle, and as you get thereon, you are feeling the bike hold your weight. You'll not fall. Put your feet on the pedals and begin cycling. As you cycle, you continue faster and faster. Your heart is racing from the much-needed exercise. You are feeling good. Your lungs start to harm, but you push yourself as you notice the wind flying through your hair. Notice the droplets of sweat cool your skin. You bought this, and you're coming to a curve within the course now. Turn your bike and follow the trail to the finishing line.

As you reminisce, you'll see people a bit like yourself competing to end, and there are a couple of behind you and a couple of before you. While exercising, take a gentle breath in and push it out forcefully.

You ought to hear a pushing sound coming from your pursed lips. Inhale and say, "I got this, I won't hand over. I will be able to succeed." you're coming to the finishing line now, but the course isn't over yet. As you cross the finishing line, you get off your bike in third place. Thanks for going!

Bring your attention now to your breath. You're breathing heavily, your heart is racing, your chest hurts, but it is a euphoric feeling. You are feeling free; you broke out of the cycle and crossed the finishing line. As you're taking a glance down your body, you notice your body has become thinner. There's a scale ahead of you on the sidelines; you've lost ten pounds. the sensation you're experiencing at this very moment is breathtaking, so you would like to undertake it again. Trust that your body knows you and what to try to. Trust in yourself that you simply will get through this.

You prepare again and wait to listen to the coach. Take a deep breath specific a count of 5 . once I count, you'll start your course. Five, four, three, two, one, and go! Let loose your breath and feel your legs carry your ten pounds-lighter body. This point is a little more comfortable than the initial round. Your breath quickens, and your heart accelerates. You'll do that.

Say to yourself

"I will complete this course. I'm strong enough to overcome any barrier that stands in my way. This way is often hard, but nothing easy is worth doing. I got this."

In front of your now's a blow-up house with a good opening. You crawl through this opening and are covered by colorful plastic balls. They're flying at you from all angles, and it becomes hard to ascertain. Soon, you're swimming through these balls moving forward. You push these balls aside, and as you search, you see another opening. "I got this,"

You tell yourself

"I will make it through, and zip can stop me now." As you reach the opening, you crawl through and are entirely on your stomach. You're during a narrow hole that you simply must army-crawl through to succeed in the top. Absorb a deep breath now. Nothing scares you. Nothing can get to you. Imagine this hole the way everyone else bullied you or picked on you. You would possibly have felt small, or enclosed, singled out, or trapped.

You have complete control, and you'll do that. You're coming closer to the sunshine at the top now. Nothing can stop you. As you reach the top of the tunnel, you leap out and begin doing jumping jacks and yell to the universe, "I did it!" You beat your fears, and you conquered the darkness, but your journey isn't over yet.

On the proper side of you, there is water on the table with a scale right next to it. You down the water and tread on the size. You notice your weight dropped another ten pounds. because the euphoric energy escapes you, you are feeling happy and delighted.

As you look before you, you see another course twenty feet away and, therefore, the finishing line at the top. Take a breakthrough now. Walk or jog at your own pace. You bought this. You've got faced harder challenges before, so you're getting to get through this one. Twenty steps later and you reach a potato sack, and five tires on the bottom laid call at a line. You jump into the potato sack, and while holding it up, you jump into the first tire hole. Take a deep breath in, and now the second tire hole. Exhale, jump into the third tire, now the fourth, and take some time. Inhale and jump into the ultimate tire.

As you leap out to end, exhale slowly. You'll feel your heart aching from the exercise. Pat yourself on the back; you're almost there. On the left side of the track, you notice weight balls that attach to your ankles and two five-pound dumbbells. You connect the ankle weights, devour the dumbbells in each hand, and appearance forward. The finishing line is ten steps away. Take a deep breath in. "I'm almost there, I won't give up." exhale and take your initiative. The load around your ankles was an equivalent amount of weight you carried at the start of the race. You notice what proportion of a difference this is often and never want to desire this again. Take another breakthrough and feel the sweat drip down the rear of your neck. Feel the exhaustion.

Now visualize your ideal weight. Let that be your motivation to continue. With every step, you become more and more tired.

Your body becomes more and more exhausted, but you do not hand over, you retain moving forward; the finishing line just steps away now. Take a deep breath in, and there's no way you're abandoning now. You're so on the brink of your ideal weight. You've got almost accomplished your goal. You hear the people on either side of you cheer you on. Yes!

You crossed the finishing line and felt that it had been all worthwhile as you step onto that scale beside you. And right before your very eyes are the numbers you've got wanted to ascertain for therefore long.

You did it! Congratulations! You're now at your ideal weight. Visualize what this seems like and absorb the thrill. Visualize what feeling you'd experience after completing your goal. Stay relaxed at this moment for as long as you'd like.

When you are ready, come to this moment. Bring your awareness to your breath. Move each finger and wiggle your toes. Feel good as you remember your visualization. You completed your goal, and you didn't hand over . that is what you'll prefer to neutralize your waking life a day. Everyone has obstacles, but you've got the willpower and now the talents to beat everyone that gets in your way. You'll open your eyes now.

Perfect Weight

"Of perfect mind and ideal weight." The terms could seem sort of fantasy to you; the sound mind and, therefore, the ideal weight. They're the realistic conditions it's possible to use as you pursue weight reduction. "Realistic?" you ask. "How can anything be 'ideal,' including my burden and my ideas about my weight?" Well, recall what we said about the facility of believing and belief. Can it serve your curiosity to desire or hope for love or money but perfection on your own? Indulge us for a few times as we clarify why you can think your mind and burden as "perfect."

Perfect weight is the weight that's ideal for you. It is the weight that's achievable and according to everything you would like and what you're able to give yourself and accept on your own. More to the purpose, your ideal weight provides you the healthy body, the body which matches effortlessly, and also the one where you're feeling great about yourself and joyful. And what're ideal thoughts? You currently have a complete thought process, and it's flawless. But there are often a couple of ideas in those typical thoughts of yours that are providing you undesirable outcomes. There is usually something you hold in your mind, possibly habits or routines, which give you adverse outcomes. However, you'll use your ideal thoughts to align your ideas to supply you precisely what you desire. You'll use your thoughts to accomplish the bodyweight you want.

In the Twinkling of an Eye Fixed

Your current body is the outcome of your ideas and beliefs. You've acted out these ideas and feelings by the way you reside, which generated your current weight. You haven't made any errors, no matter what you'll be thinking of yourself; instead, you've just experienced undesirable outcomes. These unwanted effects are an instantaneous effect of misaligned ideas and beliefs about yourself, which are your very patterns of behavior or way of life. The Self- Hypnosis Diet is all about using your ideal thoughts to align your ideas to supply you with the results you desire. You can actually use your mind to accomplish the bodyweight you want.

Now, watch the learnings have occurred in your life, which has gotten you to where you're now together with your weight. Are you able to awaken one afternoon, and there, you're using all the extra pounds? Or was it a slow accumulation with time? Or perhaps you've understood nothing else from early youth. Regardless of the situation, many factors made your body what it's today, such as:

- Food choices

- Eating customs

- The self-critic in you

- Economic history

- Emotional background

- Influence of household

- Impact of friends

- Cultural heritage

All these and several other variables were learned in your life and eventually became your beliefs, which subsequently became patterns of activity that generated your weight. We'll be more specific and notice which those aspects appear right for you in your previous years. In other words, consider what you probably did understand in your youth about eating and food.

- What sorts of grocery did your household buy?

- What meals did your parents cook, and were they typically ready?

- Do you consume food, only reception, or does one often grab fast food?

- Have you been served fresh, healthy, home-cooked foods, or did you eat mainly processed and highly processed foods, fried foods, and "junk" foods?

- What did you understand about eating mindfully?

• Have you been taught that healthful food options led to healthy bodies?

• Did anyone teach you ways you'll understand what's healthy food and what isn't?

• Were your food selections supported, which tasted or seemed great or priced less?

Examine your own socioeconomic or sociocultural roots, and see whether or not they had an impact on the way and what you learned to consume. Over thirty-five decades back, sociological research acknowledged weight issues from the working and class consistent with their intake patterns of what has been referred to as "poverty- grade foods," like hot dogs, canned meats, and processed luncheon meats.

Cultural groups even have been analyzed to know their dietary patterns and meals, like cooking with lard or ingesting a diet of high fat and fried foods, which will cause higher body fat gain. These influences can readily be accepted because they're "normal" within the group or course. Then let's take a glance at the adolescent years. During adolescence, were there any changes in your weight? As a boy, were you invited to pile more food on your plate? "Look at him, eat more! Certainly, he's getting to become an outsized guy!" (There's a telling metaphor) Or are you currently admonished to eat? When you are a budding girl, did a sensible girl take you under her wing and ask you that the marvel of menses and, therefore, the wonderment of body modifications, as an example, organic growth in body fat with the expansion of breasts and broader shoulders?

Were you conscious during puberty, wherein, unless your body improved body fat by 22 percent, it wouldn't correctly grow and make menses? Or was that "hushed up" within a clumsy improvement? It had been likely during adolescence which you heard there is a stigma regarding obese men and ladies. Spend a few minutes writing down the aspects that appear to be accurate for you in your previous years. Ponder the encounters and influences which formed your body.

In high school, the athletes at school sports have always been a wholesome weight, so are also the cheerleaders and homecoming queens.

What could ancient beliefs about your popularity and self- image have formed out of the societal interactions in high school? What did you understand about physical activity, and what customs did you produce? Have you ever been introduced to physical activity as a part of a healthy lifestyle, through family or sports outings of walks or hikes? Or was the blaring TV a traditional fixture, enticing everybody to the sofa?

Next may be a question which most of the people haven't been conscious of during their evolution. As you're growing up, was the eye of self-care supported trendy clothes, makeup, and hairstyles, or on healthy food, routine physical activity, and spiritual and intellectual nourishment? What about today? Spend a few more minutes writing down the aspects that appear to be accurate for you within the past few decades. What influences and experiences shaped the ideas, which turned within the beliefs, which become a body?

After high school, you moved far away from home. Suddenly, you do not accept as true with your family's lifestyle. Did you become more conscious of your options, or did you begin eating to detach steam? If you entered into an in-depth connection, what compromises or arrangements about food and physical activity, did you share input?

Most relationships develop from similar pursuits, like food preferences and eating styles. Within the end, the connection comprises eating routines and tastes, which are a consequence of compromise. Have your relationships encouraged smart food choices and healthy eating? Maybe you've experienced pregnancy. Are you able to learn the thanks to getting a wholesome pregnancy and nourish a healthy infant within you? Or did you add pounds?

After parturition, did your lifestyle assist you in recovering your healthy weight or inhibit it? Within the event that you simply were active during a league or sports matches, did your livelihood or family duties take priority and eliminate these fitness activities from your regular?

Did you correct your exercise and diet? Or did the load begin to accumulate? Did an accident, injury, or illness happen that disrupted a traditional physical activity that has been supportive of a healthy weight?

It's possible to notice that how you bought and to where you're now was no accident. You heard from the parents around you and, you also collated out of the environment the way to produce food decisions. The thanks to eating, and, therefore, to taking care of yourself emotionally and physically. Whether the ideas you heard were great and healthy or not so great and not so healthy, they became your own beliefs, and eventually became you and your body because it is today. Bear in mind, you didn't do anything wrong, but you've experienced the outcomes of eating and living, which are according to your ideas and beliefs.

More than the years, what's been your answer to people and their opinions about your weight loss? bad or good? Are you able to leave and buy an incredible pair of sneakers, or did you consume more to ease the psychological distress?

Maybe you even heard the latter response in your youth. Did your mom ever provide you with a plateful of food to comfort you once you felt miserable? These are learned responses, and that they are often unlearned and replaced with new answers and patterns to form your ideal weight. You ask, "Just how long does this take?" We inform you, "In the twinkle of an eye fixed ." For the minute you understand that you simply need it enough to try to anything to possess it, it's completed. You've just altered the management of highly efficient energy in you, which can be directed at deciding the way to get the result which you need: your ideal weight.

Your Perfect Mind Relearning

It isn't difficult to grasp how you bought or "heard" to weigh over your ideal weight. And it will be simple to make new decisions, to relearn new routines, and also to form new and far healthier habits. How can we learn? The simplest and most lasting learning entails repetition and practice. The most straightforward thanks to training are vital.

Pretend for a moment that you are a violinist. You're rehearsing for a grand symphony operation in NYC. Your piece includes a neighborhood of 5 pubs that's extremely hard for your fingers to perform correctly. There are two ways in which you practice. The first, which is sort of ineffective, would be to play that tough segment fast, over and over and once again, always playing the same mistakes, but trusting that your hands will play it properly

The next way is to the clinic, which can always be useful. Here, you perform the section very slowly, mindfully "teaching" your palms the thanks to maneuver, making the "muscles" ready for the acceptable moves. You are doing this steady until your palms have discovered the steps and may play the entire segment correctly and within the appropriate pace with small, if any, mindful focus.

The important thing here is that you're giving your attention to practicing correctly. By being conscious of what you're exercising, and therefore the way you're practicing it, you're studying the new patterns which are replacing the previous routines. You're practicing the action that generates your ideal weight. You, too, can create "muscle memory" by practicing mindful eating (eating slowly, chewing thoroughly, swallowing the last bite before you're taking

another bite) or maybe a more cautious, slower fork-to-mouth motion. You'll even practice an entire dining design that becomes conditioned as mind-body learning or memory, which instantly becomes intuitive. Because it will become an inherent or second character, you do not get to believe doing it.

Chapter 8

Tools for Reducing Body Weight

Stimulus Control

The skill of keeping your environments stocked healthy food choices and cleared of trigger foods that make temptation.

For many years, the man spent an intrinsic part of his life chasing down food to eat. Today during a world overloaded with food choices, food is now chasing us, and it's winning.

Fat Thinking and Stimulus Control

I always ask Shift Weight Mastery Process participants to list the environments, times of day, and trigger foods they reach for. Most of their lists aren't long, but they're explanatory!

•   Cheese once I return from work—with wine!

•   Crackers or chips ahead of the TV.

•   Eat from my boss's candy jar within the afternoon when I'm stressed.

•   Eat leftover cake within the staff room.

Nine times out of ten, when a client has had an error and increased a couple of pounds, it's because of a tempting food or a specific set of meals among the environment.

Never underestimate the facility that food— especially an interesting trigger food—has on your brain and your ability to regulate it.

Trigger foods are foods that you simply can't eat just a touch of. They tend to be a food that activates your brains got to eat more and more until the bag, box, or bowl is empty. Trigger foods also tend to be highly refined foods that contain big mouth and brain pleasers, like sugar, fat, and salt. There are exceptions to the present rule. Some people choose to spread , dried fruits, cheeses, or high-fat dairy. Any food you discover yourself circling back for or brooding about can pose a "stimulus" issue.

According to Brian Wansink, Ph.D., author of Mindless Eating, when adults are put into a state of perpetually having to decide whether or not to concede to food temptations, they get worn down and eventually concede. That's why counting on your ability to be strong and exert willpower within the presence of your favorite, fattening trigger food may be a sort of fat thinking. It just doesn't work.

Thin Thinking and Stimulus Control

Weight Masters adopt a proactive attitude with their environments instead of a defensive one. They use their minds to think on a particular level—protection. You'll cultivate thin thinking by choosing foods that are getting to be best for you in your environments and avoiding foods that challenge your weight release and maintenance.

Here are two thin thinking strategies which will make an enormous difference to your long-term weight release success:

• Stimulus-proof your environments, like your home, work, gym, car, or anywhere where you spend time and/or are susceptible to eat your trigger foods.

• Create loving boundaries together with your trigger foods.

Stimulus-Proof Your Environments

This three-part stimulus control strategy is incredibly easy in theory. Your challenge is to form it a practice.

Keep Healthy Snacks Available

You enter your front entrance after spending the last 45 minutes in traffic, and your blood glucose level is dropping as you head into the kitchen. You've got to start dinner, but as you open the fridge to tug out the salmon and salad fixings, the first things your eyes fall on are three leftover pieces of pizza. What proportion willpower does one need to assert not to stand there and erode least a couple of bites of that pizza, if not all three slices?

What if the pizza was within the back of the fridge during a covered container, and therefore the very first thing you saw was the salmon and green beans you're getting to steel oneself against dinner and a box of pea pods and cucumber slices to munch on while you cook. Because you wouldn't see the pizza, your mind isn't engaged to believe it and doesn't need to exert energy to resist it. Out of sight, out of mind, and out of mouth!

Make some extent once you shop to possess healthy snacks to succeed in for at work and reception and altogether of your environments. If you retain the healthier options upfront and simply available, your mind will stay tuned to nourishing yourself.

If a Food is Challenging You, Move It or Get and obviate It

There are a couple of ways to try to this:

• Keep challenging food out of sight. Creating a visible barrier between you and, therefore, the food sometimes is enough. I had a client who put a barrier between her and of the corn chips on the table at Mexican restaurants by placing the napkin holder and glasses to cover it. Put trigger foods in cupboards or drawers or within the back of the pantry so that they aren't in sight.

• Freeze the trigger food. This way works great for bagels, bread, cookies, and food. It removes the urge to pop some into your mouth impulsively.

• Dispose of the food. If the tactics still don't work, put the food within the garbage, and if you continue brooding about it, put the food within the trash on the road. That, my dear apprentice, is stimulus control. The rubbish disposal works well too. Remember, it's not a waste of cash if it saves you from pain and suffering. Avoiding the few hours of feeling bad about yourself is well worth the price of disposing of some trigger foods.

Stimulus-Proof Your Shopping

Millions of dollars are spent getting you to steer zombie-like down grocery aisles, putting the beautiful packages in your cart, and getting them through checkout stupidly about the later consequences to your body and your weight struggle. Don't be a pawn in their numbers game! Take back your power at the shop.

We often undermine our weight management by buying things for people at the grocery. Parents often use the excuse that "it's for the youngsters ." Two more common explanations are "what if friends come over" and "it's on sale." Shift your mind and stay focused on what you would like from the grocery. Walk by anything that you simply know are going to be calling your name later that night. Make a shopping list and stick with it!

If your Inner Rebel says, "I need to buy frozen dessert for the youngsters," but it's you who finish up eating it, expire the frozen dessert. How? Take a deep Shift Breath, connect with your thin thinking Inner Coach, and ask yourself:

•   If I buy this frozen dessert, what is going to happen to it?

- Is that frozen dessert getting to be calling my name all night?

- Is that frozen dessert getting to be for the youngsters or the guests? Will I find yourself watching rock bottom of the empty carton and cursing myself for falling for the old "it's for the kids" con again?

Love yourself enough within the moment to mention "no" to the impulse. You're doing yourself an enormous favor by setting yourself free from the cravings, the food-sneaking behavior, and, therefore, the guilt after you eat it. Just walk on by. have you ever passed the frozen dessert aisle yet? Phew!

Stimulus-proofing your environments may be a potent strategy. You'll be amazed at what proportion easier weight management is when your settings are freed from the trigger foods that cause you problems.

I am not saying that you simply need to remove all the unhealthy foods or treats from your house. I'm sure many diets don't hook you. I do know that I can have bags of potato chips sitting in my cupboard for months and that I couldn't care less. Chips don't roll in the hay on behalf me so that they don't get to leave my house. However, it's a particular issue altogether once you are talking candy and gumdrops! Those sugary candies are a trigger food on behalf of me. I do know if I even have one, I also have to eat the entire bag. So, guess what? They don't are available at my house.

If they are doing, my family is under orders to not let me know. What my mind doesn't realize won't stimulate it.

Creating Loving Boundaries with your Trigger

Foods

Life is long, and there'll be times once you want to enjoys an enjoyable treat, including your trigger foods. How does one set your mind up for fulfillment when having that treat? Make a rule together with your Inner Coach before time about. When and the way much of a gift you're getting to enjoy. That treat isn't an option at the other time. I call this strategy, "creating a loving boundary."

Alain Dagher, Ph.D., a neurologist at Montreal's Neurological Institute, conducted a study on expectation and brain activity concerning smoking. He measured the brain activity of smokers who were kept from smoking for four hours. One group was told that after four hours, they might smoke; the different group was told they needed to still abstain from smoking for six more hours. The smokers who expected the cigarette after four hours began to point out high levels of arousal, the closer their time to smoke came.

The other smokers, who didn't expect a cigarette, showed no arousal. When the brain knows that a gift or treat won't be forthcoming, it puts its attention elsewhere. Once you create a choice about something, and you're clear that boundary, it helps your mind say "no" comfortably.

Here's the way to roll in the hay step by step.

• Identify the trigger food. This way could be easy; it's the one you can't stop eating!

• Think of what one serving would be both in amount and calories. Confirm it allows you to remain within your Calorie allow Weight Release.

• Think of an environment during which it'd be safe to eat one serving. This environment is one that you simply haven't had a stimulus control issue in.

• Create a limit on how often you would possibly enjoy you trigger food during this setting. Creating a limit keeps you from overindulging or abusing the boundary.

For example, say your trigger food is a frozen dessert. If you didn't stop eating the frozen dessert until the carton is empty, our stimulus control strategy would be to stay frozen dessert out of your house. But what if you would like to be ready to enjoy its creamy goodness every once during a while? You'll create a replacement loving boundary with a frozen dessert.

For example, a loving boundary for frozen dessert could be "Once every week, and I can have a scoop of my favorite at the frozen dessert parlor."

You are giving yourself something you enjoy but during a moderate and measured way outside your environment. You'll even search the frozen dessert calories online and see that one scoop of rocky road is 170 calories. You'll make it work calorically for you on the day you have it, too. You've got the frozen dessert but still, remain within your Calorie allow Weight Release.

My Loving Cake Boundary

The frosting was my drug of choice once I struggled with my weight. At one wedding, I went back for five pieces of bride cake. Of course, I had to stay face. I didn't want the server to think that I used to be an out-of-control cake fiend. I told him that I used to be bringing the additional slices to others at my table. Little did he know that the others at my table were my Inner Rebel and her wild friends partying on cake deep inside me!

As I started my journey to weight mastery, I created a healthy and loving boundary around the cake that works on behalf of me still. I tell myself, "Cake and frosting on behalf of me isn't an option unless it's my birthday or the birthday of anyone in my immediate family."

This fundamental rule around the cake may be a perfect fit for me. For every family member's birthday, I will be able to make a cake and have an exquisite piece with extra icing. In my inner rule system, the cake isn't an option unless it's my birthday or my husband's and children's birthdays.

Create Your Trigger Food Loving Boundary

Exercise

Take a flash to fill in your trigger foods and make a loving boundary.

• Stimulus-proof your environments by removing the trigger foods that tempt you and having healthy choices available, once you aren't falling victim to high-calorie foods in your situation, it's much easier to remain consistently on target with weight release.

• Bringing healthy food into your environments and having them available for meals and snacks is different to make sure your situation is about up to assist you in succeeding.

• Create loving mental boundaries around your favorite trigger foods so that you'll have them in your life occasionally but in a controlled way. Knowing your trigger foods and creating a masterful relationship with them puts you responsible.

- Stimulus control is a crucial skill not just for releasing weight but also for long-term weight management.

APPRENTICE PAUSE: have you ever felt protective of somebody or something? Perhaps you've got cared for a little child or a pet? It's quite an intense feeling, right? Why is it that when it involves your self-care and weight, you don't step in to guard yourself? Now that you simply understand the skill of stimulus control, you'll be your protector, bringing a replacement level of self-protection to your life within the way you're taking care of yourself and, therefore, the environments you reside in.

Weight Loss Hypnosis

To start this hypnosis, confirm that you simply are during a comfortable position. Don't attempt to do that once you are driving and wait to try to it publicly, like on a bus or a plane. You are doing not skills your body might react, so it's best if you're focused on doing this reception while on your couch, or perhaps as you're falling asleep. Remove all other distractions and focus only on staying comfortable. Focus only on your breathing and hear the subsequent directions as you begin to fall under a relaxed state.

For this hypnosis, you're getting to visualize what's waiting ahead of you. Let the thoughts flow through your mind as if they're your own.

Everything that we are getting to discuss during this motivation is about you, and only you. We are getting to begin with "I" statements because these are affirmations. These are the thoughts you would like to urge into your head to rewire the way that you only are thinking towards something more positive and healthier.

I am inhaling and that I can feel myself fill with life because the air enters my body. Because it comes, I count one, two, three, four, and five. Because it exists, I count six, seven, eight, nine, ten. Counting my breath helps me to manage it. When my breathing is regulated, everything else in my body is going to be also. These processes are reliable, and that I understand that my body is capable of anything.

I have begun to concentrate on the items that I'm eating to assist me in reducing. Within the past, I used to be unhealthier and that I made poor decisions for my body.

This way has led me to where I have gained weight, and now, I feel unhappy with the person who I even have become.

I have tried to reduce it within the past. I even have considered eating foods that are bad on my behalf and that I may need also considered some unhealthy dieting methods, like crash dieting or harmful pills.

I did this because I used to be taught to hate my body. I wanted to punish myself for the shape that I had found myself in after making more unhealthy choices. I made unhealthy decisions to undertake and reduce, not that specialize in my psychological state within the process.

These unhealthy choices led me to an area of negative thinking. I feel bad thoughts about my body, which only makes it harder on behalf of me to reduce.

At this moment, I'm getting to stop this negative thinking. I will be able not to be focused on hurting or punishing myself anymore.

The only thing I care about is ensuring that I'm a healthy person. I'm focused when it involves my health and, therefore, the foods that I'm putting into my body. I care about the wealthy , but I care even more about feeling better.

I am uninterested in trying a new diet after a new diet. Each new thing I discover, I buy small hope, but it fails. It doesn't fail due to the meal plan, but due to my mindset. I buy frightened of what is going to happen once I fail, so I'd not even try within the beginning.

I am not getting to allow myself to think like this anymore. I'm only getting to be focused on positive thinking and a healthy mindset to assist within the achievement of my goals. I don't want to urge stuck within the same thinking pattern for the remainder of my life. I deserve better. I deserve entirely just hating my body.

I need to be happy from the within, which will start to point out on the surface.

I am always surprised at how hard my body works because it consistently exceeds my expectations.

Once I am sick, I'm wondering if I will be able ever to feel better, but my body does most of the add fighting things off. I'm ready to achieve great things with my body, and therefore the only reason I'd have fallen off my healthy lifestyle path within the past is that I did not see that initially.

Going forward, I'm getting to be focused on seeing the fantastic things that I'm capable of. I'm only curious about tracking the items that I even have done. I'm not focused on the topics that I'm still waiting to accomplish. I'm grounded within the "now," because that's the sole thing that matters to me during this weight loss journey.

I am centered with my body, and I'm determined to urge it to the right place. I'm not getting to try anything harmful to reduce. Instead, I'm getting to work with my body, not against it. I'm getting to use the tools that are the foremost helpful in ensuring that I reduce successfully, so I don't need to worry about it returning on later in life.

I am taking a positive path towards getting the items that I desire. I felt like weight loss took goodbye before. Often this is because I used to be tracking my progress multiple times each day. Within the past, if I didn't see results within a few days, then I might think that something wasn't right.

I understand now that this was just a mentality that was taught to me. My body works much faster than I'm ready to see, but I wont to only measure it by the items that were happening on the surface.

Moving forward, I'm only focused on measuring progress with how good I feel. Accepting this mentality alone makes me feel better already. once I am clearly focused on ensuring that my psychological state is that the most vital, then everything else seems such a lot easier.

The reason weight-loss felt love it took goodbye within the past was because I used to be impatient. I understand how time works now and that I realize that I can't track things as closely as I want to. Within a month, I will be able to see far more progress than what's seen during a day, and that I understand the difference now.

I am understanding of how I want to twiddle my thumbs, and the way this mentality will help me to reduce rapidly. If I buy too impatient, I will be able to attempt to rush a process that takes time, and it'll only make it feel longer within the end.

I am not getting to give my attention to fast weight loss. I am getting to ignore the size.

I will only specialize in numbers during a long-term sense, like monthly weigh-ins.

I am getting to be the foremost concerned with how I'm feeling mentally.

If I ignore how I feel mentally, then this may only hold me back further and keep me within the place that I'm already trying so desperately to urge out of.

I am not getting to fight against my body anymore. I'm only getting to confirm that I'm using its natural processes to reduce. Once I am often patient, it'll make the load loss feel much faster.

I am getting to keep track of my weight loss reasonably, and I'm getting to drop the unrealistic expectations that I've created for myself.

I am getting to be compassionate to myself during this process. I understand that I will be able to make some mistakes.

I have the motivation and encouragement needed within myself to form sure that I don't let these mistakes become defining moments in my life.

Each time I feel as if I even have slipped far away from a goal, I will be able to remember that it's up to me to urge back on target from an area of determination and dedication.

I am getting to be forgiving of myself for my natural urges and need to follow old habits.

I am getting to be more reliable than the person who I used to be within the past, but I also remember that they're still strong themselves.

I am focused only on living a healthy lifestyle and losing weight rapidly. I understand that thanks to making this process fast is to stay to it. There are not any shortcuts or quick fixes. This way is often a process that's getting to be a lifelong journey, but that doesn't mean I can't still see results within a comparatively close time-frame.

I understand that being patient and sticking this diet out is what's getting to help me reduce the quickest.

I accept the very fact that I cannot rush this process and need to take it because it comes. My body knows what it's doing and that I trust that it's the facility to form up for the items that I cannot control. I'm getting to encourage my body to reduce through keto and fasting, but it'll still be up to my body what proportion weight I will be able to lose and at what pace.

I will not compare my body to others anymore. I'm only focused on myself and that I know that I even have all the facilities needed to seek out success.

As I continue during this hypnosis, I'm reminded of where I'm now and where I will be able to be going next. I'm getting to count to 10, and once I reach ten, I will be able to be out of the meditation and either drifting to sleep or back within the world where I'm more focused and prepared to lose the load. My breathing remains regulated and can still plan the hypnosis has ended. One, two, three, four, five, six, seven, eight, nine, ten.

Chapter 9

How to use Meditation

Today's world is simply so fast-paced that it seems like we've no time to hamper, relax, and be calm.

Even once we continue the holiday, we take over the office and add our heads, worrying about subsequent committee meetings, a disgruntled client, or where the next deal comes from.

We think we're happy and calm, but within our minds, there are many hidden stresses, fears, worries, and thoughts going deep. Once we don't take time to relax and quiet the inner noise consciously and intentionally, tension will build up and inevitably affect the standard of our lives, and the way we affect people around us.

It needn't be like this. Meditation practice will allow us to settle down and obtain still. It helps our mind to urge concentrated and relax, helping us to deal with all the everyday stresses of a busy life.

Not Just a spiritual Act.

People typically classify meditation as being purely for religious or spiritual activities. Although many religions are correct to form reflection a part of their religious practice, it's not merely a mental activity alone. But more and more people that aren't religious accept meditation practice.

If you are feeling like life is getting a touch too hectic and leaving you stressed, then slowing down, calming, and relaxing would be an excellent time. Meditation will assist you in achieving a relaxed state you would like to ease your mind and free from stress

Meditation Advantages

Still, wondered why people are meditating? Which difference, which value does it bring back their lives? I used to be at a coffee point in my life once I started meditating and crying about the loss of my friend. I started meditating on my counselor's suggestions as to how to assist and ease my worries and continue my wellbeing and core strength building cycle.

A lot of individuals have various reasons to meditate. Once you are contemplating, what was your reason to meditate? To an outsider, if you meditate, what they see you are doing is sit down, maybe cross- legged on the ground, watching some extent within the distance or sit together with your eyes closed.

How does this, practicing meditation, influence your state of mind? Yet most of my students in yoga and meditation swear that meditation for quarter-hour each day is that the neatest thing they will do to offer them the strength, motivation, and compassion they have to try to whatever they have.

Meditation is a few mental activities that have significant health benefits both for the mind and, therefore, the body. Meditation can help relax the mind, establish a more concentrated state, and enhance the functioning of the brain.

Medical evidence suggests that meditation practice appears to elicit A level of physiological relaxation: decreases in vital signs, slower heartbeats, and faster breathing, and other biochemical improvements can occur also.

•	Meditation reduces the consequences of many chronic illnesses, like a heart condition, cancer, and diabetes.

•	It helps and soothes chronic pain, anxiety, and migraine.

•	Meditation helps improve the role of the system and also prevents binge eating.

•	The asthma attacks offer considerable relief.

•	Reduces lactate within the blood, minimizing depression and anxiety.

•	Meditation has been documented to also help in lowering cholesterol.

•	Reduces muscle tension, and therefore the system is relaxed.

•	It assists in building self-confidence.

•	It helps monitoring aggressive mind.

•	Increases synchronization between brain waves.

- Removing unhealthy habits helps.

- Assists in the creation of intuition, imagination, and concentration.

- It improves the power to recollect and enhances memory retention.

- Enhances sleep habits and assists in eradicating insomnia.

Meditation is the process of thought intensely for a short time or relaxing one's mind. This fact will be wiped out silence or with the help of singing and is completed for a spread of reasons, ranging among religious or spiritual motives to how to induce relaxation.

Meditation has, in recent years, grown in popularity in our modern, eventful world as to how to alleviate stress. It's also emerged scientific evidence that meditation is often a valuable tool within the

fight against chronic diseases, including depression, a heart condition, and chronic pain.

This ancient custom has many various aspects to it.

If you're curious about trying meditation but do not know where to start, here's another list of sorts of practices:

Breaking the trance: the two athletes (runner within the hypnotic state and idol) were taken back to their forum, and therefore the athlete returned to rest on the bank before either awakening secure and refreshed or drifting off to sleep and awakening afterward feeling refreshed, relaxed and efficient.

Having a recording that takes you thru these stages is often an accurate idea because you'll hear it and do not got to believe recalling the things. You'll use it before bedtime if you've got trouble sleeping and fall asleep to sleep afterward. If you would like to be a touch more sophisticated, you'll also help to feature some background music.

I hope you've got enjoyed this chapter in which you'll find the suggestions useful. Hopefully, it all is sensible, but please get in-tuned if you've got any questions, and we'll do our greatest to elucidate and help.

Training your mind takes time and practice, so work with it and provides it time. It's almost like physical training to urge stronger as you recognize and obtain won't to new, more useful ideas and feelings. Good luck, and have fun

How Can I Remain Motivated to Lose Weight?

The most critical aspect of making constant and virtually infinite inspiration is linked with all the explanations you would like to lose weight.

Confine mind the broader sense of weight loss for you, like your health needs or how it can positively affect you each day, and therefore the people around you, like your family and shut friends.

Specialize in clear, observable, achievable, timely, and practical objectives. Make short but attainable goals first to seek out enjoyment and fulfillment in constant progress towards achieving long-term goals of weight loss.

Have a clear, rational mind of not being too easy or too hard on yourself to succeed in the objectives by keeping the arrogance and frustrations going distant.

Find people around you with an equivalent drive as you are doing, and you're always encouraged and challenged to continue pushing for similar goals.

When you can keep these continually in mind, you'll find that you simply will feel more motivated and determined to figure through obstacles and circumstances toward achieving your long-term goals.

Methods of meditation

Conscious Meditation

It is easy to urge trapped during a loop of spinning thoughts — beginning to believe a laundry list of activities to try, ruminating about past events, or potentially future situations — and practicing mindfulness may help. Yet, what exactly is attention? It is often described as a psychological state that needs to be fully working on "the now" so that, without judgment, you'll understand and acknowledge your thoughts, feelings, and sensations.

Mindfulness Meditation

Mindfulness meditation may be a sort of mental preparation that helps you to hamper thoughts of running, abandoning of anger, and relax both your mind and body. Mindfulness methods can vary, but a meditation on mindfulness generally involves breathing exercise, imagination, body and mind awareness, and relaxation of the muscle and organ. Practicing meditation with mindfulness doesn't require props or planning (no need for candles, essential oils, or mantras, unless you enjoy it). To urge going, all you would like maybe a comfortable sitting spot, three to 5 minutes of spare time, and an attitude that's freed from judgment.

Mindfulness meditation is the method of getting your thoughts fully present. Knowledge involves being mindful of where we are and what we do, and not being too sensitive to what's happening around us.

One can do reflective meditation anywhere. Some people wish to sit during a quiet spot, close their eyes, and specialize in their respiration. But at every stage of the day, even when driving to figure or doing chores, you'll prefer to be conscious.

You track your thoughts and feelings while practicing mindfulness meditation but allow them to move without judgment.

Transcendental Meditation

Transcendental meditation is an important technique whereby an individually defined rhythm, like a word, sound, or short phrase, is repeated during a particular way. It's exercised twice per day for 20 minutes while sitting comfortably on the brink of the eyes.

The hope is that this system will allow you to settle into a deep state of relaxation to realize inner peace without attention or effort.

Directed Meditation

Directed meditation, often also mentioned as guided imagery or visualization may be a meditation technique during which you create mental images or scenarios that you simply find calming.

Guided meditation is among the foremost standard methods of meditation employed a day by many people. During this post, we'll explore guided meditation and the way to try it.

In the purest form, guided meditation may be a sort of meditation where the individual is guided on every step of his daily practice. Someone directs you right from the primary level of sitting during a meditative pose to the ultimate phase of completing the meditation. What occurs is that in meditation, an educator or mentor provides step-by-step guidance about what to try to. It's an ancient method of conveying directions for meditation to pupils. In older times, this system has been wont to teach meditation during a group. Nowadays, because of technological development, we do not need a guru's physical presence to steer us in meditation.

We will hear a master's direct guidance using pre-recorded CDs or DVDs and conduct our meditation practice. Within the absence of any meditation master professional CDs / DVDs, you'll record the instructions of guided meditation from a book in your voice then play them afterward.

Furthermore, if anyone doesn't have the potential of a voice recorder or a DVD player, during a session, he may ask his friends or relatives to talk about the written meditation instructions orally. This way, we will use the advantage of guided meditation but with none technological assistance.

However, I still believe that the utilization of a pre-recorded CD or DVD for guided meditation is that the best way for guided meditation because it removes the necessity for an individual to be physically present near you to read the instructions. It also allows you to cash in of controlled meditation, even when you're alone.

Guided instructions for meditation are often of varied varieties counting on the methods the teacher imparts. A number of the foremost collective meditation techniques utilized in guided meditation are Vipassana. This meditation involves visualization of the cycle of breathing, visual imagination, mantra recitation, a meditation on dancing, a meditation on prayer and meditation on mindfulness, etc. the simplest thanks to using guided meditation is to concentrate to a master's live guidance. If this is often not feasible, then the second-best option is to record in your voice the written instructions of meditation then hear it in your meditation practice.

Usually, this phase is directed by a guide or instructor, thus "driven." it's also recommended that you simply use as many senses as possible, like a scent, sounds, and textures, to elicit calmness in your relaxing region.

Vipassana Meditation

Vipassana meditation is an ancient sort of Indian meditation that suggests seeing things as they're. Quite 2,500 years ago, it had been taught in India. Conscious meditation movement has origins during this practice within us.

The purpose of meditation with vipassana is self-transformation through the examination of oneself. This way is often accomplished to make a deep connection between mind and body by careful attention to the sensations within the body, the sustained interconnectedness results in a cheerful account, crammed with love and compassion.

Vipassana is typically taught during a 10-day course during this tradition, and other people are expected to follow a group of rules all the time, also as for abstaining from all intoxicants, telling lies, cheating, sexual intercourse, and killing any animals.

Loving Meditation on Compassion (Metta Meditation)

Metta meditation also called meditation on loving-kindness, is that the practice of guiding good wishes towards others. Those that practice reciting similar words and phrases will elicit warm-hearted sentiments. This way is often commonly found also in meditation on mindfulness and vipassana.

It's usually wiped out a pleasing, relaxed position while sitting. After a couple of deep breathes, you slowly and steadily repeat the following words. "Just let me be happy. May I be fine. Let me be free. May I be calm and at ease". After a period of guiding this loving- kindness to yourself, you'll begin to imagine a loved one or friend who has supported you and repeat the mantra, this point replacing " I " with" you." As you continue the meditation, you'll bring back mind other members of your family, friends, neighbors, or people in your life. Practitioners are often encouraged to think about individuals who are having trouble with them.

Finally, you finish the meditation with the quality mantra: "Let every being be happy everywhere"—a meditation on the Chakra.

Chakra is an ancient Sanskrit term that will be traced back to India and translates into a "cycle." The chakras ask the energy and spiritual force centers within the body. It's believed there'll be seven chakras. Every Chakra is during a different part of the body, and every one of them features a corresponding color.

Chakra meditation consists of relaxation techniques that aim to bring balance and well-being to the chakras. Any of those techniques provides the visual depiction of any chakra within the body and, therefore, the corresponding light. Some people can like better to light incense or use crystals, which are color-coded for every Chakra to assist them to focus during meditation.

Meditation Yoga. The yoga practice has its roots in ancient India. There is a right sort of yoga classes and designs, but all include performing a series of postures and guided breathing exercises designed to encourage flexibility and relax the mind.

The poses require balance and a spotlight, and practitioners are encouraged to concentrate less on distractions and remain more at the instant.

Which meditation style you select to undertake depends on several factors. Once you have ill health and are new yoga, tell your doctor what method would be right for you.

Ways to Promote Meditation into Your Life

Treat yourself to ice cream? Are you stuck within the motorway? A lover in wait? Here's the way to make these moments a meditation.

Which one considers harder: in sleep, taming your monkey mind, or doing overtime only to take a seat still every day? Either way, fear not: by merely integrating meditation into your daily activities, you'll quickly reach a relaxed state of mind.

•   Do this you would like to try to. If it's a hiking, walking, cooking, or painting, while we concentrate wholeheartedly on our favorite things, time stands still. Mysteriously, our stream of emotions, stories, and dramas fall away. Submerge yourself during this one fantastic thing, and do not attend to those pings! Then keep an eye fixed on your feelings. Calmer, then? Feeling happier? Congratulations — you've just completed a meditation on the influence of this moment. That's so simple.

•   Nurture nature yourself. Life doesn't sort of a popular dietary supplement, with people hiking a day happily.

And almost anytime you go outside, you'll quickly practice meditation. As you adapt to the first rhythms of nature, your breath and thoughts hamper to match the gentle march of mother nature.

• Only making yourself like your ten-year-old self and observing the clouds overhead will transmute stress. Extra credit if you think about heart types blowing down the shadows.

• Wait, not, meditate! You meet a lover, and she or he is delayed — again. Seek a smartphone meditation rather than dalliance tweeting and texting. Indeed, there's an application for that! Plug your earbuds, and you're all of a sudden, engaged during a 10-minute session that's oh-so-soothing. By the time you're done, bet you, your friend arrives — which you welcome her with a warm embrace rather than the "late- again" eye-roll.

• Time to fly. If you're caught in traffic, now isn't necessarily the time to "be one together with your fellow riders" and surrender blissfully. You would like a serene diversion. Try a mantra meditation set to make super chill music (I am a serious DJ drez fan) or invent your own ("I am love, I'm light") and obtain lost as you walk down the lane.

• Think with pillows. You'll turn sluggishness into a sublime meditation once you have a wee little bit of resistance to roll out of bed within the morning — plus, you get to remain a touch longer! Lie still, and watch your scarcely conscious feelings. Once we bear witness, "I don't need to travel to work" becomes "I see struggle — and I am fine thereupon ." bonus points for adding a purpose to your day — sort of a decision to embrace your emotions or a love offer to friends and family.

• Eat your favorite food, drop-dead. Step into the kitchen together with your oh-so-spiritual self and scoop a little helping of frozen dessert or anything tickles your buds. I'm going with cherry Garcia from ben & jerry, so work with me: consider lifting this funny little mound on your lips.

Consider the temperature, taste, and smell as cherry and chocolate bits gradually slip down your throat. This ancient tradition of mindful eating is both an important rite of contemplation and an incredible way of expressing appreciation for our abundance. Ben & Jerry: namaste!

• Meditation, meditation, and yoga, and more. Truth: Whether you're trying to touch your toes or improve your handstand, the one reason we're doing yoga is going to the super- end- of-class climax moment once we drop into a meditation savasana. It's the physical poses that allow us to urge into that dark, still space in our minds. Regardless of what degree or lineage you practice, all postures cause a state of meditation that's all-spacious.

Daily Meditations and Habits

Now I'm close to taking you on a journey of visual imagery and relaxation to a far-off place. Enjoying vibrant and compelling images, you'll hear powerful and definite statements that will endorse many feel-good affirmations, which will improve your perception of yourself and improve your overall wellbeing.

We tend to show food whenever we are stressed in life. When problems overwhelm us, most folks tend to stress and eat, and then we experience a cycle of guilt and regret. In time, this cycle can impact how we feel about ourselves.

During this guided meditation, you'll remember the way to feel good and understand your connection to food. During times of stress, you'll study letting go of tension and to experience all that's natural and instinctive.

The experience of this guided meditation is going to be enhanced if you discover yourself a cushy and ventilated spot.

Ensure that there's no disturbance from anything or anyone for thirty minutes.

You need to settle on an edge to lie or even sit comfortably for the duration of this exercise. It's a realistic idea at this point to unplug or mute your phone.

Now, you would like to shut your eyes and steel oneself against a deep sense of relaxation and wellbeing. Remember that this is often some time, and embrace the chance to flee from the stressful world you reside in. You'll now relinquish all the unhealthy habits and learn to spice up your guiding force.

At this particular moment, there's nothing that you simply got to worry about. You're asleep, and you're safe. You'll allow the tensions of the day to dissipate so that you'll connect with your inner self. Together with your eyes closes, breathe deeply and slowly through your nose then exhale through your mouth. Once you inhale, you're taking all that's good and positive about this world into your body, and once you breathe, you're letting go of all tensions and unnecessary fears.

Now, inhale again. Inhale slowly through your nose to the count of 4. One, two, three, and 4.

With your lungs now filled with oxygen, hold your breath for 2 seconds.

One and two.

And now exhale slowly through your mouth. You would like to exhale to the count of 4.

One, two, three, and 4.

When you inhale, you'll slowly feel your diaphragm expand once you feel the air enter your lungs. Inhale until you feel like your lungs are filled with air.

Strive to regulate the exhalation of air and confirm that you simply steadily exhale you would like to continue this cycle of rhythmic breathing.

Inhale to the count for four.

Hold your breath for a count of two. Exhale your breath to the count of 4.

You can resume breathing normally, and you'll feel all the strain in

your body slowly dissipate.

Acknowledge that your body is now beginning to feel more relaxed. Your arms and legs will start to feel heavier.

Relax the strain in your lower back, middle-back, and your upper back. We frequently tend to store tension in our shoulders. Learn to release it. Once you are abandoning the strain you are feeling in your body, you'll feel your body relax.

Elongate your neck so that there's space between your ears and shoulders. Once you slowly elongate your neck, you'll feel the mattress you're lying on or the chair that you quietly are sitting on support your back.

Now, scan your body and check if there are any areas of tension left. If you feel that there are some, then you would like to tighten the muscles in those areas and abandoning deliberately. Once you are doing this, you'll feel your body relax. You'll feel the strain leaving your body.

Now, you would like to travel into a state of deep meditation.

To do this, you would like to continue the rhythmic breathing exercise.

Imagine that you simply are now standing during a beautiful meadow with soft rays of sunlight falling on you.

You can see an arched doorway that's carved into a rising cliff.

Your surroundings look quite peaceful, and you are feeling good.

You can see golden sandy beaches behind you and azure blue skies above you.

Now, you're slowly making you thanks the arched doorway. The door is within your reach; the wood feels warm under your fingers. As you trail your fingers across the door, you'll feel a way of pleasure and wonder as you imagine what lies behind the door.

To enter, you would like to stay your mind hospitable the wonders that lie ahead. Reach out and slowly turn the handle of the door.

As you emerge, you'll see a lush and delightful, bright-green rainforest.

The air feels fresh and pleasant under the cover, and therefore the welcome change from the sun-drenched beach a couple of moments ago.

Take a deep breath then exhale to embrace this sense of peace.

As you begin to steer forward, you notice a trail that leads through this beautiful rainforest.

As you search, you'll see the glimpses of a gorgeous blue that's speckled with soft, cotton-like clouds.

Continue scanning the sky all around you.

You are surrounded by majestic mahogany trees that reach up tall towards the zenith.

You marvel at the dark brown bark of the trees that seems to possess a delightful sweet odor.

Space is restricted here, but you're grateful for the narrow trail that leads you thru this place of natural wonder.

You can hear the melodious chirping of birds all around you. It seems like the forest has to wake up around you.

All of this appeals to your senses, and you're ready to experience nature in its pristine form.

Consider if you strip back your own life and are to measure more naturally what proportion better will you are feeling.

Only a little percent of sunlight can penetrate onto the ground of this rainforest. So, you progress further call at the wilderness, and you'll see the flashes of exotic blue butterflies dancing around you.

You can hear the melodic sound of running water within the distance, and you are feeling compelled to maneuver towards it.

As you're taking within the wonder of the beautiful nature all around you, you progress towards the larger expanse of the forest area that results in a weak stream of water.

There are natural stepping-stones that lead you to a pool of water that appears crystal clear. Green plants surround the pool of water.

You walk closer to the pool, and you notice plants with colorful berries all around.

There are several fruit-bearing plants, and everything looks rich, exotic, and tempting.

You take a bite of those delicious berries, and you'll feel a burst of flavors.

The berries taste delicious, and you'll feel this deliciousness because it makes its way right down to your stomach.

Your body feels energized.

Some stones are present around and across the water, and as you walk, you begin to become one with nature.

You notice carefully carved out steps higher within the rocks, and you begin to climb.

The climb is sort of easy, and it feels almost effortless.

You feel an exquisite stretching in your muscles once you grip the rocks for balance.

There is no fear of falling.

As you grip the rocks and make your high, you are feeling slimmer, stronger, and toned.

You feel exactly how you would like to explore and the way you would like to be.

You pull yourself up higher and better . you're slowly progressing towards the cover.

You can feel the air become purer.

You start to inhale pure oxygen and abandoning of any tensions you're holding onto.

Your 'normal' looks like it's miles away.

You consider how good you are feeling at this moment. You still make your way towards the cover.

You don't need to fear the peak since it's safe, and you can't fall.

You don't feel tired or exhausted. During this world, you are feeling fit, healthy, and knowledge of an abundance of energy. You're determined to urge to the highest and see the view from the highest of the cover.

Imagine walking up through these steps until you reach the ultimate stage and you reach the top of your journey.

You reach an outsized platform that overlooks the tops of the trees.

Directly across from you, there's a rock face with water cascading down. The water is frothing abreast of its way down the rocks, and therefore the sight is mesmerizing.

You can reach up and touch the clouds. You'll feel the clouds around you.

The sky looks beautiful.

Visualize these pleasant sensations that course through your body during this instance.

You experience a way of relaxation. Every inch of your being feels good.

Take this moment and visualize yourself stretching.

Stretch up high and feel the wonderful sensation as you elongate your spine.

Now, keep your back flat and move forwards and down. Allow your body to relax forward. Imagine the incredible stretch you'll feel within the ends of your legs- there's no pain, just a joyful sensation of movement.

Your spine starts to relax, from your lower back through to your neck as you lift your arms. Your neck and your head relax as you lie on the mossy platform.

Keep your arms behind your head and your elbows wired. Engage your core muscles and check out to lift your shoulder and your head towards the clouds above.

Visualize yourself lifting and interesting those core muscles while you attract your stomach and tighten your abdomen. All of this causes you to feel so good.

Now start to relax once more.

Start to consider your breathing. Inhale as you open up your chest and exhale slowly.

It is time that you simply start to feel good about the person you're. It's time to feel content and embrace pure inner peace. Here during this rainforest, you're liberal to explore and be the person who you would like to be.

Let go of any unhealthy eating habits, and it's time to be kind to your body and to nurture and protect your body.

Repeat these affirmations to yourself and believe each word.

Believe in the message and, therefore, the power these words need to change your life.

I will change my perception of my body. I recognize my self-worth.

I will change my eating habits so that I see my food as fuel and nutrients instead of food.

I will exchange binge eating for breathing techniques and guided visualization.

I will start exercising and changing how I look and feel.

I will create an activity diary and plan the way to embrace exercise. I can face my inner fears and make the required positive changes.

Sit quietly for a flash and let these affirmations become a neighborhood of you.

It is time to feel positive about your life.

It is time to face any weight issues head-on. You have the facility to try to so.

At any time, you'll return to the present rainforest and knowledge of the wonders of nature. You'll find your inner strength and inspiration during this shelter.

You are centered, and you keep the sensation of peace and wonder.

Enjoy the instant and, therefore, the feeling of harmony that you simply experience.

Breathe in then out.

Retain your sense of peace and your desire to nurture your body. Breathe in and out.

You will change your association with food. Breathe in and out.

Slowly open your eyes on the count of three.

One, two, and three.

Now, you're back in your reality.

Stretch your body slowly and still take deep breaths. Realize how good you are feeling during this moment.

Remember your desire to enhance your fitness and your wellbeing.

Return to the present shelter of yours whenever you would like to enhance your health.

You can use this system anytime you are feeling tensed or nervous. Whenever you are feeling stressed, rather than reaching for a packet of chips or the other food, you'll do this simple exercise to calm your mind. You'll breathe thanks to a stress-free life.

Cleansing Relaxation Meditation

This meditation is all about focusing on becoming relaxed and cleansed. One of the best ways to achieve this kind of feeling is through the use of music.

Make sure that you are somewhere comfortable. You need to be in a peaceful and distraction-free zone in which you can close your eyes and focus on nothing but feeling the air come in and leave your body.

One of the reasons why we struggle to lose weight is that we are so stressed. Stress can lead to stress-eating and cause your body to hold onto weight that it does not need. Worse, it can alter your hormonal levels.

You are focused now on reducing stress because this means that it will be easier for you to lose weight. There is nothing else that you are concerned about other than becoming more relaxed.

You are centered; you are focused. You are at this moment; you are prepared for whatever might come your way. You are not concerned with anything other than relaxing and becoming more peaceful.

Feel it as the music beats to a rhythm. There is a slight beat, no matter what it is that is being played. Everyone who listens to this will find a different meaning to the tunes. Everyone who partakes in the process of listening to cleansing music does so for various reasons.

It will always help everyone to relax. Though we all have different things that we use this music for, it still helps us to become more and more at peace. Calmer and calmer. More and more relaxed.

Start to focus on your breathing now. Breathe along with the music. Count for at least five while you are breathing in and then five as you are breathing out.

Breathe in for one, two, three, four, and five. Breathe out for six, seven, eight, nine, and 10. Feel as you breathe in how the music enters your body. Your body is like a musical song as well. Your heart is like the drumbeat that is always pounding.

Your brain is like the conductor that tells everything how it should sound. Your blood, your muscles, and your organs – they make up the rest of the instruments. Your body is a beautiful chorus, and you are a melody traveling through life.

You are a perfect being, relaxed, calm, and at peace, and you are one with the earth. You are one with the music. You start to feel it come in and out of your body.

This music can change the way you feel, and this music is in control of your emotions. It will affect the way you operate.

It is helping you to feel better and more relaxed. It is bringing you closer and closer to being at peace. It is bringing you closer and closer to being centered and focused.

You are feeling lighter and lighter, and the stress is drifting away. As soon as you start to let go of stress, you will begin to release yourself from the heavyweights that are keeping you back. The more focused you are on your breathing pattern, the easier it is for you to feel relaxed. The quicker you focus on peace, the more weight you will lose.

Each time you let go of stress, you are letting go of some of your weight. Every time you focus on being more at peace, you are feeling healthier and healthier.

You feel it as the music spreads to every part of your body. It starts in your mind. It stimulates your brain so that you are focused on relaxing and nothing else at that moment.

It soothes your heart. It reminds you that you are not alone. It makes you feel better, and that spreads everywhere else.

The music keeps you motivated. It keeps you cleansed.

Cleansing is an important part of your weight-loss journey. Your body is always working to clean itself. Your body is focused on how it can rid itself of toxins and bring in the things that are good for it. Your breathing is one way that your body is consistently working to cleanse itself.

Your body is always cycling in new air and getting rid of the old. It does the same thing with food as well. It brings in new minerals and nutrients and gets rid of the toxins that it does not need. You drink water to help cleanse your body. It is always working on its own to keep you as purified as possible.

The cleansing processes help you to feel more at peace. You feel like a new person, and you are constantly given second chances. It is never too late to start over.

You are feeling your body become more and more cleansed now. Then you are feeling lighter and lighter, more relaxed. You are becoming a new person. You are starting over. You are starting fresh. You are relaxed. You are focused. You are at peace.

As we count down from 20, you will exit this mediation. Continue listening to cleansing music to bring in the peace that you need to lose weight and maintain it. It will be easier to lose more weight when you manage to focus on cleansing.

Twenty, 19, 18, 17, 16, 15, 14, 13, 12, 11, 10, nine, eight, seven, six, five, four, three, two, one.

Chapter 10

Dealing with Food Addiction

Until now, you've got been taking note of multiple reasons for weight gain. Some may say that overeating causes weight gain; some may believe that it's due to hormonal issues. Some may say that the lazy routine is that the explanation for obesity. We cannot deny them. All of them are correct. But if you dig deeper, you'll find causes of most problems in your head, including overeating and other purposes that are mentioned.

How does a food addict's brain differ from a naturally lean female brain? This section describes the most characteristics of the differences within the mind, especially in food addicts.

We are crazy about food. -We usually force us to eat. -We need more menu to be full. -We often suffer from hunger. -We respond more strongly to food references. -Emotional imbalance causes brain hunger in us.

Functional Resonance Imaging (fMRI) uses the magnetic properties of blood to work out which area of the brain is most active when a topic experience a specific event. Neuroscientists can measure brain activity when food addicts are exposed to food labels, eat delicious foods, or eat certain foods. "It's like training," explains Dr. Ashley Gerhardt. "When you train a specific muscle, blood flows into that area. The brain seems to be working a similar way, and you'll track which area of the brain receives the first blood."

fMRI consistently shows that the convergence zone for sensory information is that the prefrontal cortex, associated with reward stimuli, particularly primary reinforcement factors like food. To elucidate the neurobiological mechanisms by which weight, mood, and age affect the appetite response, Dr. Gerhardt presented healthy, average weight, obese adolescent and adult women with color photographs of foods with different fat content and caloric density while undergoing fMRI (high reward vs. low reward). She shows that food-addicted women skilled highly rewarded foods within the same way drug addicts answer drugs.

Dr. Bart Hoebel, originally from Princeton University, he was one among the primary to review a mouse for sugar addiction. He showed that each drop of sweet they swallowed increased the amount of dopamine. Almost like human addicts, Hoebel's rat sugar developed a hypersensitive dopamine receptor that was hyperresponsive to a spread of medicine, and its changes were long- lasting. Even after a month of self-discipline, the taste of sugar stimulates the rat to become addicted.

In a similar study, in Birmingham at the University of Alabama, Dr. Mary Boggiano found out that a food attack in rats elicits an equivalent pleasing receptor within the brain that drug addicts are stimulated once they ingest drugs. Dr. Boggiano's oleo-conjugated rats have long-term changes in endogenous opioids within the brain and become abnormally aware of delicious food.

And if this chou tastes nearly as good as sex, it's no coincidence. The dopamine reward system is that the way we feel good and is related to obsessive gambling, drug abuse, and sex. Food satisfaction results from several equivalent neural signals and pathways that regulate orgasm. As a result, many neuroscientists have begun to record that obesity, eating disorders, and even healthy appetite resemble addiction. "Repeating dopamine over and over is what drug abuse does," says Dr. Hoebel. "This causes you to wonder if food may have addictive properties.

Food gives you a discreet physiological response within the same way that drug consumption gives you an enormous response," says psychiatrist Walter H. Kaye, director of the Eating Disorders Program at the University of California, San Diego. The drug takes over the food reward. "Drugs are addictive because they open the way for appetite.

Like other drug therapies, food therapy is an effort to realize the dopamine levels required by all addicts. During a 1954 study identifying amusement centers, two McGill University researchers, Dr. James Olds and Dr. Peter Milner, documented the consequences of dopamine. During this study, rats were ready to push the bar to electrically stimulate the amusement center or push the bar for food. Dr. Olds and Dr.

Milner said electrical stimulation of rats to an amusement center is more rewarding than eating. The experience was so satisfying that the hungry rat ignored the food for pleasure the electrical impulse from the entertainment facility gave her. Some rats stimulated the brain quite 2,000 times an hour for twenty-four consecutive hours. Most mice died on an empty stomach.

Heroin and cocaine addicts also happen to ditch eating and lose tons of weight while taking the drug. This fact explains why you get dopamine fixes from other sources. The primary stage of affection, all the activities that we discover so enjoyable, we don't eat much and forget to eat! Poisoning is high dopamine, not food. If this mechanism fails, we find yourself eating an excessive amount of food, hooked into repairing dopamine.

So, that's how you overeat. You are doing not eat because you wish it, but you eat because you're compelled to consume. Now we'll check out sorts of overeating.

Lightning Source UK Ltd.
Milton Keynes UK
UKHW020643240521
384271UK00011B/781